"I can't wait to recommend this book to everybody I know. An absolute 'must read' for anyone with digestive discomforts or those who desire total health."

Ann Louise Gittleman, PhD, CNS
Best-selling author of *Fat Flush Plan* and *Gut Flush Plan*

"Finally, someone has the guts to head off the impending acid-blocker crisis . . . Martie Whittekin has made a very complicated subject understandable and reveals the true answers to solving the real problem and at the same time improving your overall well-being."

Fred Pescatore, MD
Best-selling author of *The Hamptons Diet*

"So you think you need an antacid or acid-blocking drug? Read this book and you'll understand why your problem is not likely to be solved by these drugs. Find out the truth behind your symptoms with healthy ways to prevent them—while improving your overall health and well-being at the same time!"

Hyla Cass MD
Author of *Supplement Your Prescription: What Your Doctor Doesn't Know About Nutrition*

NATURAL ALTERNATIVES TO NEXIUM, MAALOX, TAGAMET, PRILOSEC & OTHER ACID BLOCKERS

SECOND EDITION

What to Use to Relieve Acid Reflux, Heartburn, and Gastric Ailments

MARTIE WHITTEKIN, CCN

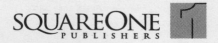

SQUAREONE
PUBLISHERS

The information and advice contained in this book are based upon the research and the personal and professional experiences of the author. They are not intended as a substitute for consulting with a health care professional. The publisher and author are not responsible for any adverse effects or consequences resulting from the use of any of the suggestions, preparations, or procedures discussed in this book. All matters pertaining to your physical health should be supervised by a health care professional. It is a sign of wisdom, not cowardice, to seek a second or third opinion.

COVER DESIGNER: Jeannie Tudor
IN-HOUSE EDITOR: Ariel Colletti
TYPESETTER: Gary A. Rosenberg

Square One Publishers
115 Herricks Road
Garden City Park, NY 11040
www.squareonepublishers.com
516-535-2010 • 877-900-BOOK

ISBN 978-0-7570-0210-6

Printed in the United States of America

10   9   8   7   6   5   4   3

CONTENTS

This book is dedicated to those who want to be healthier and feel more vibrant—especially those who believe in supporting the body's normal function, when possible, through gentle, natural means.

ACKNOWLEDGMENTS

Any of us today who write about natural health are, as they say, standing on the shoulders of giants. It would be impossible to name all of those who contributed one way or another to this book. The following is a humble attempt to name (in alphabetical order) just a few: Jeffrey Bland, PhD; the late William Crook, MD; Russell Jaffe, MD, PhD; Doug Kaufman; James LaValle, PhD, ND; Don Mannerberg, MD; Michael Murray, ND; Fred Pescatore, MD; Joe Pizzorno, ND; Doris Rapp, MD; William Rea, MD; Sherry Rogers, MD; Melvin Werbach, MD; and Jonathan Wright, MD.

These brilliant professionals have contributed personal research, analysis, clinical experience, and critical thinking. Moreover, they made science accessible and were powerful advocates for safe and effective natural methods—often in the face of skepticism, bullying, and personal sacrifice. Each has had an important impact on my career and enduring enthusiasm for natural medicine, which has greatly benefited my family, my clients, my listeners and now, hopefully, my readers.

Teachers never get enough credit, so I'd like to recognize two that greatly affected my life: My science teacher Mr. Collier inspired me to be curious about how and why things work, and Mrs. Ann Ackerman, my high school English and Journalism teacher, methodically taught me better ways to express myself. (I will send her a copy of this book, but hope she has retired her red pen.)

I'm grateful to my loving and patient husband, Bill, who put up with my seemingly endless absorption in this project and even helped prepare meals so that we didn't starve. (However, I do think the situation may have allowed him uninterrupted opportunities to watch sports.)

CHAPTER 1

THERE IS A DRAMATICALLY BETTER WAY

*"Inflamed tissues hurt for a reason. It is nature's way of
enlisting your brain to help in solving the problem."*
—SHERRY ROGERS, MD

If you frequently have searing pain and/or pressure in your
midsection, you may not care a great deal whether it is called
heartburn, acid indigestion, gastritis, gastroesophageal reflux
disease (GERD), acid reflux, gallbladder disease, or an ulcer.
After all, your main concern is likely to be reducing the pain as
quickly as possible, regardless of its name. It is certainly no
wonder that many millions of sufferers resort to acid-blocking
drugs for symptom relief rather than considering the actual
cause of the problem, the potentially lethal risks of the standard treatments, or safer alternatives.

This path of least resistance, however, can be hazardous.
Consider the following:

• The directions for acid-blocking drugs state to take them for
only fourteen days or, at most, only a few weeks. According to
the producers of these medications, a doctor's guidance is
required if they are going to be taken for longer periods of
time. Yet many users do not heed this advice, which is intended to prevent serious side effects that can be caused by long-
term use. Even physicians seem to have become casual about

those limitations—perhaps because drug reps hint at longer term safety and/or because the longer term health losses aren't easily connected with the medication.

• It is likely that the stomach acid these drugs systematically block is not the actual cause of your pain. Rather, the acid can actually be useful—even life-saving—for you.

• The pain may be caused by a minor structural issue that won't be addressed by the drug but can be solved without surgery. It is to your benefit to logically address the problem rather than mask the symptoms.

• Blocking stomach acid actually fosters the growth of bacteria that cause gastritis and are associated with GI cancer, pneumonia, and even the dreaded methicillin-resistant staphylococcus aureus (MRSA).

• Some of the current well-intentioned standard medical advice may cause more harm than good. For example, most doctors warn patients away from alcohol and fats. However, moderate consumption of alcohol and good fats may actually help the stomach. On the other hand, the over-consumption of certain inflammatory fats, refined sugar, and flour is a major cause of acid reflux, but these products are not typically included on the list of foods of which to be wary.

• Acid reflux can be caused by certain medications such as the ubiquitous statin cholesterol drugs.

• There are dietary supplements proven to heal the ulcers that are caused by common pain relievers like aspirin and Motrin.

• There are dietary supplements and simple techniques that can relieve acid-related symptoms, repair the underlying problems, improve digestion, and reinvigorate the body's overall health.

The very idea of acid-suppression is relatively new, and some of the research casts doubt as to whether the way we are using the medications is healthful. This book will explain causes of common stomach pain. Some of these causes may be surprising to you. The standardization of medical schools and medical practice too often means that the search for "a second opinion" only results in the patient being given what is essentially the same opinion twice. This book offers second opinions that are meaningfully different from those typically given. It also offers treatment options—natural approaches that avoid the many serious side effects of the acid-blocking drugs that tend to be prescribed so routinely.

These natural alternatives not only address both pain relief and the root cause of your grief, but also improve your overall digestion and offer what may seem, at first, to be unrelated fringe benefits. After all, improvements in digestion and GI function can greatly improve everyday life by lifting depression, improving sleep, boosting energy, alleviating joint pain, enhancing immune function, normalizing weight, eliminating migraine headaches, and even making skin look younger. There are also dramatic benefits of improved digestion and assimilation, such as protection from fatal diseases and a reduction in the impact and progression of autoimmune diseases.

A few decades ago, many of us giggled at Alka-Seltzer commercials, which went "plop, plop, fizz, fizz." This remedy was promoted for relieving occasional digestive discomfort from overindulging ("I can't believe I ate the whole thing") or making a bad menu selection ("Mama mia, that's a spicy meatball"). Today, it is estimated that 50 million Americans suffer chronically from some type of digestive pain and ask for increasingly more potent drugs for relief from this pain.

Unfortunately, this pain is not merely an annoying discomfort. Heartburn's more severe cousin, gastroesophageal reflux disease (GERD), is linked with serious damage to tissues and even with esophageal cancer—the fastest rising malignancy in the United States. (From 1975 to 2001, the rate of occurrence of esophageal cancer grew approximately six-fold in the United States. It carried a mortality rate that increased more than seven-fold.[1]) Chapter 3 will investigate the shocking but very real possibility that the cause of this cancer, as well as gastric cancer, may be the long-term use of the acid-blocking drugs, rather than the GERD itself! At the same time, the survival rate for gastric cancer is 23 percent in the United States—but 60 percent in Japan.

As you will see in Chapter 2, each diagnosis has distinct characteristics, but for simplicity, I will often lump acid-indigestion, gastritis, heartburn, GERD, and other similar disorders under the general label "heartburn." This is because the underlying causes of the conditions, the drug therapy, and the benefits of the natural remedies are so very similar. Much of what we will discuss as we talk about restoring balance even applies to ulcers and gallbladder problems.

The term "heartburn" is a misnomer. The "burn" part is accurate enough, but the pain certainly isn't in the heart. It isn't even in the stomach. The pain comes from the *esophagus* (also called the *gullet*)—the muscular pipe leading from the throat to the stomach. Like all physical symptoms, the pain is akin to a red warning light on the dashboard of your car. When acid-blocking drugs are used for longer than a few weeks, they do little more than turn off this light. This, unfortunately, allows us to remain unaware of or ignore the real problem—which is not a deficiency of drugs and is, therefore, usually not treated by the medication.

The fundamental problem is that tissues which are not supposed to be in contact with stomach acid are being exposed to it. A healthy stomach is well protected by mucus against the burning effects of acid digestive juices. But sometimes that protective barrier can become depleted or infected. Pain, gastritis (stomach inflammation), or ulcers can result, allowing the raw tissue to come in contact with the acid and react painfully. The esophagus, on the other hand, has no protective mucus because digestive acid is not supposed to enter this passageway. Therefore, it hurts when acid reaches it. This signals that there is a problem with the mechanism that is supposed to confine stomach acid to the stomach. Once the normal barrier is malfunctioning, digestive juices can reach as far as the throat, which can cause a persistent sore throat and cough. In extreme cases, the liquid can reach the mouth and erode tooth enamel. These fluids may contain bile, which originates below the stomach and produces a very strong bitter/acidic taste when these fluids are belched up.

But *why* are these digestive juices able to reach these areas? The problem is usually that the *lower esophageal sphincter (LES)*—the valve between the esophagus and the stomach—does not tighten as it should after food has passed through it and into the stomach. The problem is *not* that our stomachs make acid. Our stomachs are supposed to make acid. You will see that the acid-blocking drugs—the go-to medical treatment for heartburn and a variety of other digestive problems—do not address, or even claim to address, the underlying cause of the pain. When used properly and for short periods of time, these medicines can provide temporary relief while the damaged esophagus or stomach tissue heals. It is easy to see how doctors can fall into the trap of using acid blockers for most stomach complaints since the presenting symptoms of low acid and excess acid are virtually identical. However, long-term use of acid blockers may actually make the real causes of heartburn worse.

Heartburn can be caused by a variety of factors and affected by variables such as genetics and environment. We will look at the most common causes of this pain, which include those on the following list. Some people have more than one of these interrelated conditions:

- Low stomach acid

- Insufficient digestive enzymes

- Bacterial infection

- Overgrowth of yeast

- Food sensitivities

- Hiatus hernia (a structural problem in which the stomach pushes up through the diaphragm)

- Poor food choices

- Bad habits

Mainstream medicine advises people not to lie down for two to three hours after a meal. This is good advice because it reduces the chances of having a painful episode and will further the tissue's healing. However, this practice does not address any of the root causes on the list—and yet addressing these fundamental causes is important not only for achieving a long-lasting solution to heartburn, but also to promote overall health. They are explored further in several of the later chapters.

You may have thought that the first item on the list, low stomach acid, was a typo. Despite being counterintuitive, this is not a mistake. It only seems that way because we have been brainwashed to think of acid as bad. Insufficient stomach acid is one of the major causes of heartburn and a number of other seemingly unrelated symptoms. At least half of older people with heartburn actually have too little stomach acid. This decreased amount of stomach acid is something that often occurs as part of the aging process. A deficiency of stomach acid can also occur for other natural reasons or can be induced by medication. Regardless of the way in which it occurs, this depletion can cause a great number of health problems.

Stomach acid performs many crucial functions in the body. It is, for example, the first line of defense against allergens and disease-causing invaders such as bacteria, viruses, and fungi. This protection occurs even between meals. (Naturally, this makes it a problem that proton pump inhibitor acid suppressors may, as they claim, block acid for twenty-four hours a day.) Acid insufficiency can lead to bacterial overgrowth and may account for the increased incidence of potentially fatal pneumonia seen among patients taking acid-blocking drugs.

Stomach acid is also required for the absorption of some vitamins and several minerals that are needed in hundreds of critical bodily functions. One startling example is magnesium. Magnesium deficiency is a common cause of sudden death from heart arrhythmia—and the body's uptake of this mineral is reduced when stomach acid is blocked. Remember, too, that this is only one of many examples of the important roles stomach acid plays in your health. Therefore, the logical conclusion for your overall health is not to cancel the production of your stomach acid but to instead fix the problem that is preventing the acid from remaining where it belongs.

In this book, you will find out how to determine what is wrong and how to fix the pain. You will also learn methods to improve the effectiveness of your digestion. Depending on your particular situation, the answers may actually be pretty simple. However, many people suffer from refractory (doctor-speak for "stubborn") heartburn due to low stomach acid, an overgrowth of harmful bacteria or yeast, or a hiatus hernia. Although these problems are a bit more challenging to address, there are natural ways to control them. There are also safe natural choices for pain relief while you are working on the bigger issues. The goal of this book is not just to stop your pain and improve digestion, but also to improve your overall well being and energy!

The reason I can set such a lofty goal is that the root cause of your digestive problem may also be causing other, seemingly unrelated symptoms. Fixing the foundational problems and restoring your natural balance brings relief in the short term but also pays huge dividends in a wider range of long-term health issues. Don't be concerned if the options for determining cause and selecting treatment seem a little overwhelming at first. In the conclusion, I will outline, step by step, how to create a plan.

I hope to encourage you to take charge of your health and think outside the acid-blocker bottle. That change of view should be applied to a great many conditions because drugs taken under ideal conditions, as prescribed in hospitals, kill over 106,000 people each year.[2] If we are to make a dent in the sickness care crisis that threatens to bankrupt our country, both doctors and patients must start thinking about diseases and symptoms in a new way.

This book is not intended to replace competent medical care. In fact, it would be great if you shared a copy with your physician if he or she is open to new healing ideas that, although supported by scientific research, aren't publicized through the usual pharmaceutical industry-dominated channels. If, on the other hand, your doctor refuses to discuss alternatives, it may be time to seek out a second opinion from a professional with a different type of training and a more collegial outlook.

CHAPTER 2

WHAT THE HECK IS THIS PAIN?

*"It's no longer a question of staying healthy.
It's a question of finding a sickness you like."*
—JACKIE MASON

There is an interesting yet disturbing trend in today's society. Most people today seem to *expect* to be sick, to have some kind of disease. Most blood tests don't evaluate our health, but rather look to see just how sick we are. Our doctors don't examine us to figure out why we feel so darn good but to see if they can weave our complaints and test results into a syndrome (a pattern of symptoms) for which there is not only a Latin name, but also a recommended pill. Television commercials even turn stages of life into diseases and want you to suggest their pills to your doctor. At social gatherings, you may find yourself feeling left out if you are the only one without high cholesterol, a blood sugar problem, or acid reflux!

The truth, however, is that most of our bodies are capable of feeling great and operating well until a very advanced age. Yet to achieve our potential, we cannot simply resign ourselves to poor function and blindly control symptoms with medications. That may be the norm, but the practice puts us on a very slippery slope toward more disease and disability.

Most (and perhaps all) drugs have side effects. Too often, patients are then advised to take medication for those side effects and then more medication for the second-tier side effects. Drugs for digestive issues are not an exception to the rule. If you go to a doctor with virtually any digestive complaint, you will most likely exit the office with a prescription, probably for an acid blocker. Yet "acid-blocker deficiency" is not an actual diagnosis. Even when an acid-suppressing drug *is* the ideal initial step, these medications are only proven safe for use over a matter of weeks. To heal the root cause of the complaint and get off the medication, your problem needs to be given an actionable diagnosis. After all, you can't make an informed decision regarding your treatment until you know exactly what is going on!

As you will see, the conditions listed below overlap a great deal in their symptoms and descriptions. With some, the difference is just semantics—different names for the same thing. Others are different stages of the same problem. Also, some are different problems but are actually caused by the same underlying factors and can be treated with the same drugs—or better yet, remedied with the same natural approaches.

It is always important to ask your doctor questions and stay informed regarding your health. Some conditions require special treatment and a few can require emergency care. Arm yourself with knowledge of the potential disorders so that you can assist your doctor in making a proper diagnosis.

CONDITIONS THAT CAN CAUSE STOMACH PAIN

• *Acid indigestion.* See GER, GERD, Heartburn, or NERD.

• *Acid reflux.* See GER, GERD, Heartburn, or NERD.

• *Barrett's esophagus (BE).* Long-term acid reflux or GERD can lead to this condition, in which there are abnormal cells in the esophagus that in turn may become cancerous. This cancer is the fastest growing malignancy in western countries. There is also an increased risk of death from other causes among those affected with BE. Although the reason is as of yet unproven, it may be that the health and nutrition deficits that cause BE also contribute to the increased risk of pneumonia and heart disease. On the other hand, it may also be that the long-term use of the acid-blocking drugs prescribed for most BE patients is to blame.[1] After all, the use of acid blockers is associated with an increased risk of pneumonia and a decreased ability to absorb nutrients that are important for cardiovascular health. Although the preponderance of recent studies seem to be looking for genetic links to BE, one study found the intake of fruits and vegetables (but not supplements) to provide a significant preventative effect against BE.[2] Another showed that multivitamins and antioxidant dietary supplements helped prevent the progression of BE to cancer.[3]

• *Dyspepsia.* An umbrella—and somewhat old-fashioned—term that refers to pain or an uncomfortable feeling in the stomach. The pain can be intermittent or constant. It can be gnawing or burning, and can include burping, nausea, and bloating. "Non-ulcer dyspepsia" refers to this pain when the problem has not yet created a lesion in the mucosa.

• *Erosive esophagitis.* See Erosive reflux disease.

• *Erosive reflux disease (ERD).* A condition in which the inflammation of the esophagus has become serious enough to cause erosion (eating away) of the tissues. Risk factors for ERD include being male, consuming alcohol, having a body mass index (BMI) of over 25, and having had hiatus hernia. Many sufferers also have a history of eradication of *Helicobacter pylori*—a bacterium that causes stomach irritation and ulcers.[5] (Yes, this relationship does seem counterintuitive. Complete eradication of *H. pylori* is also associated with an increase in cancer of the esophagus. See Chapter 6 for more information.)

• *Esophagitis.* This term is used to describe any inflammation, swelling, or irritation of the esophagus. Esophagitis can occur when a person suffers from the conditions of acid reflux, ERD, GER, GERD, or NERD; receives radiation treatments or medications; or is infected with the herpes simplex virus (HSV). A form of this condition can also be caused by *Candida albicans* yeast. Candida esophagitis is commonly thought to be a problem only with the elderly and in individuals with severe immune deficiency.[5, 6] However, it may also be caused by the inhaled steroids used for asthma[7]—or even by acid-blocking drugs.[8,9] According to other sources, it is actually common if one looks for it.[10] If your main problem is consistent pain on swallowing, you could have infectious esophagitis.

• *Gallbladder disease.* Everyone has some gallstones. The situation becomes problematic when a gallstone blocks the bile duct or the gallbladder ruptures. Consider that your gallbladder may be the cause of your pain if you have chronic constipation, feelings of fullness, and/or gas or nausea, and especially if the distress tends to worsen after a fatty meal. The pain is often severe and is usually located under the breast bone, on the right side, or in the upper middle of the abdomen. It can radiate to the back or below the right shoulder blade, and becomes worse when breathing deeply. Nausea, vomiting, chills, and shaking may occur when the condition is very serious. Acid blockers will not resolve gallbladder inflammation or do anything for gallstones.

• *Gastritis.* An inflammation of the stomach membranes. Gastritis can be caused by many of the same factors that cause heartburn, such as medications, including non-steroidal anti-inflammatory drugs (NSAIDs), and the bacteria *H. pylori.* Symptoms include belching, abdominal bloating, nausea, and vomiting, as well as a feeling of either fullness or burning in the upper abdomen. This condition, especially when associated with an infection of *H. pylori* bacteria, can progress to stomach cancer. Acid blockers are routinely used along with antibiotics in the treatment of the bacterial infection. Whether or not blocking the acid is necessary or even helpful in that case will be discussed in Chapter 6.

• *Gastroesophageal reflux (GER).* A condition in which digestive fluid from the stomach travels upward into the esophagus. Although most people periodically regurgitate some stomach acid and fluid into the esophagus, GER occurs when it happens often enough and the exposure is prolonged enough to irritate tissues and cause pain.

• *Gastroesophageal reflux disease (GERD).* A chronic form (occurs two to three times a week or has lasted for at least three months) of GER. The digestive fluid in sufferers of GERD can cause an erosion of the esophagus. Once this erosion has begun, the condition becomes ERD. Nearly one-third of people with heartburn have visible evidence of erosion. Oddly, people with GERD may or may not feel heartburn. Extended and severe cases are associated with other symptoms such as halitosis (bad breath), painful swallowing, persistent sore throat, hoarseness, excess saliva, or even erosion of tooth enamel. GERD is most likely to occur in people over the age of fifty. It appears that hiatus hernia and elevated blood sugar are important causative factors that are not being adequately addressed. GERD is called GORD in some countries because they spell the name of the gullet "oesophagus." See also ERD.

• *Heartburn.* Pain or feeling of burning just below the sternum (breastbone). The pain can be felt in the chest, throat, or jaw but is actually coming from the esophagus. It may be accompanied by chronic cough or sore throat or even confused with asthma. The pain can come immediately upon swallowing or up to several hours after the meal. Fluids such as stomach acid, pepsin, and even bile can come up so far that they are actually tasted. Only one-third of people with heartburn show erosion of the esophagus, but most heartburn will likely progress to that stage if action is not taken.[10] Heartburn can affect children. (It is worrisome that drugstores now stock Tagamet for children as young as two years old.) The condition also commonly affects pregnant women because of abdominal pressure and increased levels of the hormone progesterone, which has a relaxing effect on the LES (the sphincter that separates the esophagus from the stomach). Yet acid-blocking drugs have not been tested for use during pregnancy, so natural remedies should be considered as treatment. See also GER, GERD, and NERD.

• *Indigestion.* A lay term for an unsettled feeling in the stomach after meals. Indigestion may include some nausea or bloating. It may be a result of any of the conditions listed here.

• *Nonerosive reflux disease (NERD).* This is a form of GERD in which the tissue has not yet begun to erode. A Korean study found that the risk factors for NERD are quite different than those for ERD. According to this study, NERD sufferers are more likely to be female, have glucose levels over 126 milligrams per deciliter (mg/dl), smoke, have a stooping posture at work, and have used antibiotics.[11] A Hong Kong study showed that NERD patients showed a higher prevalence of *Helicobacter pylori* infection and irritable bowel syndrome (IBS) than those patients without NERD.[12]

• *Parasites.* These are organisms that can cause many symptoms, including digestive complaints such as diarrhea, nausea, heartburn, vomiting, gas and bloating, foul-smelling stools, weight loss, gastritis, fever and chills, headache, constipation, blood or mucus in stools, and fatigue. Many people falsely believe that these pests are only of concern when we drink unclean water while camping or traveling outside the country. In reality, they can be transmitted by pets, by children, in food, and by restaurant personnel who do not properly wash their hands. Alternative medicine doctors often test for parasites. On the other hand, conventional doctors rarely consider parasites unless the patient presents with a stubborn case of diarrhea. For more information on parasites, read *Guess What Came to Dinner* by Anne Louise Gittleman, PhD.

• *Ulcers.* A sore characterized by dead tissue. Pain from an ulcer may be relieved temporarily by eating. It may come on two or three hours after eating, or occur in the middle of the night. In his book *Ulcer Free!*, Georges M. Halpern, MD says, "A sharp, constant pain between the base of the breastbone and the navel is the classic symptom of a stomach ulcer, but not everyone who gets an ulcer experiences pain in this area." He also says that the more conclusive but ominous sign is blood in vomit or stool. Other possible symptoms include unexpected weight loss, poor appetite, bloating, burping, nausea, and vomiting. Ulcers can be silent but often show up as stomach discomfort forty-five to sixty minutes after a meal or during the night. If you have any inclination that you may have an ulcer, get checked out as soon as possible. Ulcers are treatable, but can be extremely dangerous if left untreated. As many as 9,000 people a year die from ulcers. *H. Pylori* and non-steroidal anti-inflammatory drugs (NSAIDs) are leading causes of ulcers. Fosamax, Glucophage, and corticosteroids can also cause ulcerations. Treatment usually includes acid-blocking drugs, but the ulcers tend to return when these drugs are stopped unless the precipitating causes have also been addressed.

• *Zollinger-Ellison syndrome.* A rare condition, it involves *excess* production of stomach acid caused by a tumor in the pancreas or small intestine. It is characterized by pain, vomiting, and diarrhea. This is one of the few conditions in which the body produces too much stomach acid.

You should definitely be checked out by a doctor if you are experiencing any of the following: trouble swallowing, hoarseness, the feeling that food is stuck in your throat, frequent vomiting, coughing up blood, very dark or bloody stools, unexplained weight loss, anemia, getting full quickly, an abdominal mass, or jaundice (yellowing of the skin and eyes). Pay particular attention to the presence of these symptoms if you have a history of peptic ulcer disease or gastric cancer. Any of these symptoms can indicate serious tissue erosion or even a tumor, and being uninformed will *not* help you get well. Another overlap in symptoms is with ovarian cancer. The Mayo Clinic website includes a summarization of recent studies that identifies possible clues to ovarian cancer, which is treatable but notoriously difficult to diagnose in its early stages. Females who have digestive distress that is constant rather than intermittent and who also have "abdominal pressure, fullness, swelling or bloating, urinary urgency, and pelvic discomfort or pain" fit the profile and should be evaluated if the abdominal symptoms do not go away with digestive treatment.

Mainstream medicine rather naively considers that once you have GERD (by any of its names) you will always have it. That conclusion is consistent with the typical practice of dealing principally with the symptoms rather than discovering and healing the root causes. When patients get better after taking acid blockers, the doctors' simplistic view that acid was the problem is reinforced. But since acid blockers do not address the actual problem, the patient may have to take the initiative to discover and correct it.

Your doctor wants to help you but the best results are obtained when you are educated, prepared, and an advocate for yourself. (Office visits are typically not much more than ten minutes and much of that time will be filled with computer entries and various interruptions.[13]) Be observant of all your symptoms and make a list. Don't settle for a prescription without a systematically derived diagnosis. A specific diagnosis will allow you to much more effectively explore and evaluate conventional and natural options for treating your condition.

Ask your doctor to check you for the adequacy of your stomach acid if you have problems with some of the following. (Other symptoms are described in Chapter 4, as are the appropriate tests and remedies.)

• You have osteoporosis or osteopenia. (This one alone is a reason to have your doctor run a test for stomach acid because dietary intake of calcium in the United States is the highest of any country, so there is usually another explanation for your bone loss.)

• Your fingernails are thin and peeling or have ridges along the length of the nail.

• You can eat only a small amount at a time.

• The feeling of being very full lasts long after meal.

According to the University of Virginia Health System, you may want to ask for a test for *H. Pylori* bacteria if you experience some of the following symptoms:

• Dull, gnawing pain, which may occur two to three hours after a meal, comes and goes for several days or weeks, occurs in the middle of the night when the stomach is empty, or is relieved by eating.

- Loss of weight without dieting   • Burping
- Loss of appetite   • Nausea
- Bloating   • Vomiting

You have probably noticed that a lot of the symptoms for the different conditions that can lead to heartburn overlap. Also, the type of tests administered for the symptoms vary

Case Studies

The benefits of the natural methods to control acid reflux are not just theory. They have been proven effective time and time again. The following case studies involve real people, although their names have been changed. Look for the similarities, rather than the differences, between your case and those that follow. They may encourage you to develop a new way of thinking about health problems.

Charlie

Charlie is a cabdriver who, at the time of my cab ride with him, had been on Tagamet for years because of acid reflux. He had recently been married and visited his bride's native country. There, they ate only fish, rice, and fresh vegetables—and he had had no heartburn. Despite this, Charlie had never thought of recreating that diet here. He was quite eager to do so after we talked. Although I was unable to follow up on his progress, I have no doubt that it would work for him.

Ruby

Ruby, an intelligent executive, had developed acid reflux about the same time as she was diagnosed with type II diabetes. Typical of today's high speed, insurance-driven medical offices, her doctor did not attempt to determine the cause of her heartburn (or, for that matter, her diabetes). She was sent home with a prescription for Nexium.

A year has passed since that time and Ruby has greatly improved her diet by cutting down on refined carbs; eating more salads, fruits, and vegetables; and walking every day. These changes have improved her general health, her acid reflux, and her diabetes. Ruby has almost completely weaned herself off the acid blocker.

Rebecca

Rebecca is a sixty-five-year-old woman with a hiatus hernia. Her doctor advised her to raise the head of her bed and take the proton pump inhibitor Protonix. After a year, the doctor added a second daily dose because the original one was no longer enough.

In my opinion, it is completely unnecessary for Rebecca to be on a PPI, let alone for her dosage to be raised. Why experience the side effects of a medication when an actual solution is possible? The hernia should be fixed by one of the non-invasive methods described in Chapter 9. Because of her age, it is likely Rebecca will also need a combination digestive aid and perhaps other supplements to undo the damage done by taking the drug for an extended period. Unfortunately, Rebecca did not take my recommendations and was still taking the prescription when we last talked.

Max

Max, who owns a manufacturing plant, developed a consistent sore throat and experienced acid reflux every night after he went to bed. His doctor prescribed the PPI Protonix and his pain went away. Two years later, Max was still on the medication—which has only been studied and approved for use for a few weeks—and it was no longer controlling his pain, which had worsened over time.

When Max came to my office, I questioned his eating habits and discovered that, for the past few years, Max ate a bowl of ice cream at 9 PM every night. Eating that late caused digestion to start working right before bedtime—which is not good for digestion or sleep. He was also inviting a host of potential problems related to milk and sugar, including unbalancing his protective probiotics. The Protonix stopped the acid, but also lowered his defenses. It turned out that a parasite, Giardia, had slipped through and caused an infection. With this knowledge, Max rid his body of the parasite, stopped eating ice cream so late in the evening, and now lives without the drug.

Mike

Mike is a tall and sturdy thirty-year-old. He had pain that extended from his midsection to between his shoulder blades. An endoscopy revealed three ulcers and a hiatus hernia. He didn't want to have the hiatus hernia surgery because he had seen that it had taken a long time for his uncle's stomach muscles to heal after they were cut in his hernia surgery. Mike was also discouraged by the fact that the uncle's hernia came back after a few years. Because of his weariness regarding the procedure, Mike opted to stay on Prilosec. He was lucky to have a doctor who made some excellent recommendations regarding his habits, such as giving up sodas, not going to bed too soon after dinner, and eating more slowly. Unfortunately, after a year on Prilosec, Mike's pain came back. At that time, he was finally correctly diagnosed as having gallstones—even though he had previously been told he was too young to have this condition. His gallbladder was removed. Today, Mike has to be fairly careful about what he eats and when he lifts weights, but he is able to do so because he is at least aware of the problem.

We see many more gallbladder surgeries than we did years ago. I suspect that this increase is related to the rampant use of acid-blocking medications because there are many indirect ways in which low stomach acid can affect gallbladder function. Mike's gallstones may have been caused by his use of Prilosec. His related health problems may have been entirely resolved if he had been aware of the non-surgical remedy for hiatus hernia that is discussed in Chapter 9. Regardless, he put all my advice into action and I have no doubt he will continue to improve.

Jan

Jan had Graves' disease (an autoimmune overactive thyroid condition). Treatment for this condition was to kill the thyroid with radioactive iodine and put her on a synthetic thyroid hormone called Synthroid. She began experiencing heartburn after this treatment, and her doctor prescribed Nexium. Jan stayed on Nexium for about five years. During this time, her doctor increased her dose more than once. She is able to skip taking her dose for one day, but is in too much pain by the second day to work out without taking it. Her heartburn subsides somewhat if she avoids greasy foods and doesn't eat late at night.

Although Jan is large boned and of Mediterranean descent—two reasons why she should not be prone to osteoporosis—her bones are thinning. She is now taking Evista for that. She is also on a statin drug for high cholesterol, a diuretic for water retention, and an antidepressant.

If Jan had been my client, I would have attempted to find the cause of her original thyroid condition. I believe it may have been due to an iodine deficiency. It is certainly noteworthy that she and her husband acquired an autoimmune disease at the same time. They could have been exposed to the same environmental element or given the same antibiotics for some shared infection. Now that her thyroid is destroyed, she does need supplemental thyroid hormone and likely still needs iodine supplementation. However, although Synthroid is the most commonly prescribed thyroid drug, many of my colleagues and I have found that it is often not nearly as effective at relieving symptoms as the natural Armour Thyroid (which is also by prescription). I think there is a very good chance that the water retention, depression, and elevated cholesterol symptoms are all due to insufficient thyroid activity, and Armour may have resolved these issues. The underactive thyroid may also have caused her heartburn, as Russian research showed that an under-performing thyroid is often followed by GERD and even hiatus hernia.[14] The statin drug could also be responsible for the heartburn. I hope I've given Jan enough to think about and that she will be able to stop taking Nexium. One potential side effect of Nexium is bone thinning, so getting off of Nexium may also allow Jan to get off of Evista. A case this complex needs to be peeled back one layer at a time like an onion.

Jan's situation of being on six medications is shocking and worrisome but not at all unusual. The average American her age is on just as many. From there, most people will typically be put on even more medications in order to counteract the side effects of the previous ones. It is often up to patients to exert pressure on physicians to get to the bottom of the issue and reduce their medication load.

widely—and the exact same condition might even be given a different label by different medical specialists. The only uniformity is that physicians are generally trained to prescribe acid-blocking drugs for most of the conditions listed. The next chapter will detail the potentially harmful side effects of these medications as well as how to recognize the effects as quickly as possible in order to limit the damage. The following chapters will help you explore the possible root causes of your acid reflux so that you can treat the condition rather than the symptoms. Regardless of your diagnosis, much of the information in this book can help you because it is fundamental to good digestion and general health. At the very least, it will help you achieve better results while on the program agreed upon by you and your doctor.

CHAPTER 3

IS THE "CURE" WORSE
THAN THE "DISEASE"?

*"Half the modern drugs could well be thrown out the window,
except that the birds might eat them."*
—MARTIN H. FISCHER

Before considering whether the "cure"—acid blockers—is worse than the disease, we have to acknowledge that acid blockers are *not* a cure. These medications simply shut off stomach acid production to relieve the painful symptoms of heartburn and temporarily stop further tissue erosion while the previously damaged tissue is allowed to heal. But even the drug manufacturers themselves don't claim these products cure the problem that started the heartburn cycle. (There are some medications that use a different approach. These are discussed starting on page 184.) It is up to the doctor or even the patient to figure out what started the symptoms so that the cause can be treated. Otherwise, the drugs are simply changing the clock on a time bomb that will continue to tick.

We also must recognize that in most cases acid blockers are not actually prescribed to treat diseases. More often they are given to patients suffering from garden variety heartburn and/or acid indigestion, which are, rather than diseases, symptoms—a way for our bodies to alert us to a problem.

Therefore, a more appropriate (although less catchy) question than, "Is the cure worse than the disease?" would be, "Are the drugs that distract us from our body's cry for help better or worse than doing nothing?" This is a question that must be answered on a case-by-case basis.

As you have read, one of the major problems with our drug-centered system of medicine is that most doctors are not trained to dig for and correct the root causes of ailments such as digestive distress. Even those that have the knowledge and desire to treat fundamental origins of disease are hamstrung because the prevailing insurance reimbursement structure does not allow much time for a doctor to analyze a number of variables and evaluate your habits, let alone teach you new ones. As Sherry Rogers, MD, says, our current system applies pressure to "medicate instead of educate." Most doctors, when looking in their tool bags, see only the prescription for an acid-blocking drug. Of course, since the initiating factors are not addressed, the heartburn problems linger—and the prescription pad utilized again and again—sometimes for years on end.

The overuse of acid-blocking drugs has greatly worsened over the years. As patents on blockbuster prescription acid-suppressing drugs have run out, many companies have been able to get their products approved for over-the-counter (OTC) sale, so that a prescription isn't necessary. Cutting doctors out of the loop in this new self-service scenario makes it even less likely that the root cause of heartburn will be addressed. The acid-neutralizing and acid-blocking pills have now become a way of life for too many consumers.

Acid-blocking medications are touted as safer than many other drugs because, during the pre-approval studies, it was rare that anyone had an *immediate* life-threatening problem. However, the packages all instruct the consumer to use the medicine for only fourteen days; if symptoms persist past that point, the insert advises the consumer to see a doctor. The manufacturer is, therefore, limiting its risk by warning to use the product temporarily—while promoting the drugs as for "frequent heartburn," which implies a continuing problem and usage. Not surprisingly, untold numbers of consumers ignore the warning. Instead, they use these drugs for a much longer period of time, without realizing that the side effects may worsen the longer these medications are taken.

PROTON PUMP INHIBITORS

Proton pump inhibitors (PPIs) are a popular new class of drugs. They effectively block the production of acid and bring symptom relief for a lot of heartburn sufferers. Examples include Nexium, Prevacid, Prilosec, Protonix, and AcipHex.

The economics of these meds are mind numbing. In 2005, the top five brands generated a collective total of $13 billion in sales. Prilosec was a blockbuster cash-cow drug manufactured by AstraZeneca. When its patent neared expiration, Astra-Zeneca tweaked the molecular structure to produce Nexium. Is the new version more effective? That depends on whom you ask. Is it more expensive? Absolutely. Prilosec is now marketed through Procter & Gamble and available over the counter in a lower dosage.

In reality, the medicines may not be as effective as first believed in dampening the symptoms. A Harris survey showed that many users continue to have symptoms even while taking a PPI. Up to 75 percent of users take over-the-counter acid relievers as well.

The following effects of these medications should be carefully considered before the drugs are used. Additionally, please keep in mind that pregnant and nursing women are advised by the manufacturers against taking PPIs due to lack of applicable safety data.

Short-Term Side Effects

Although each medicine has its own slightly different profile of side effects, the class as a whole has been associated with the following adverse effects. Keep in mind that these are only the *published* side effects of the drugs. Typically, these were discovered in studies conducted before the products received Food and Drug Administration (FDA) approval and are printed in very fine print on the package inserts and in advertising. Due to economic necessity, the pre-approval studies are of very short duration. Therefore, these don't include the more elusive—and generally more dangerous—long-term effects, some examples of which are discussed beginning on page 28.

Frequent Side Effects of Proton Pump Inhibitors

- Abdominal pain (It is interesting how often one of the side effects of a medicine is the very symptom for which the drug is prescribed.)

- Constipation
- Flatulence
- Diarrhea
- Headache
- Dry mouth
- Nausea

Less Frequent Side Effects of Proton Pump Inhibitors

- Aggravated acne
- Apathy
- Aggravated arthritis
- Back pain
- Aggravated asthma
- Bladder infection
- Aggression
- Blurred vision
- Agitation
- Chest pain
- Allergic reaction
- Confusion
- Anemia
- Constipation
- Anorexia
- Coughing

- Cramps
- Depression
- Dizziness
- Earache
- Fatigue
- Fever
- Fibromyalgia
- Flu-like disorder
- Generalized swelling
- GI candidasis
- GI hemorrhage
- Goiter
- Hair loss
- Hallucination
- Heart arrhythmia
- Hepatitis
- Hiccups
- High blood pressure
- Hot flashes
- Impotence
- Increased sweating

- Insomnia
- Kidney disease
- Liver disease
- Menstrual disorder
- Migraine
- Pancreatitis
- Rash
- Sinusitis
- Sleep disorder
- Taste loss
- Thirst
- Tinnitus
- Toxic epidermal necrolysis (a life-threatening dermatological condition)
- Tremor
- Vision problems
- Vitamin B_{12} deficiency (a problem discussed in Chapter 4)
- Weight decrease *or* increase

Long-Term Side Effects

Unfortunately, the FDA does not require drug companies to study long-term effects, and the industry has no incentive to look for reactions beyond those required by regulation. Although the companies must report to the FDA serious complications that they observe or that are reported to them, it is often quite difficult for consumers or even their doctors to notice an association between a drug and a problem that develops later—and it is even more difficult to *prove* the cause/effect relationship. The inset on page 30 describes one such situation in which the FDA found that the causal relationship could not be sufficiently determined.

Robert Eli, medical researcher and corresponding author for the journal *Medical Hypotheses*, wrote an intriguing article linking several studies that implicate the use of PPIs with increasing the risk to stomach cancer. (Interestingly, the article also cites studies pointing to benefit from the herb, ginkgo biloba, in reducing the risk of that disease as well as helping to protect against ulcers and reduce the pain of gastritis. We'll look into that further in Chapter 11.) Hopefully, more research will be done to explore this possible connection.

One university study showed that long-term PPI users were 2.6 times as likely to suffer a hip fracture than those who did not take these medications long term. Additionally, the study found that the more medicine the participants used, the bigger the risk.[1] This may occur because the suppression of stomach acid interferes with the body's the absorption of calcium and other nutrients involved in bone building. On the other hand, it may be because these drugs also upset the body's natural pH balance and up-regulate parathyroid production. Parathyroid is the hormone that is involved with one phase of normal bone remodeling. It may not occur until years after the PPI is first utilized, but a hip fracture can have tremendous negative impact on the life of an elderly person and many times ultimately proves fatal.

PPIs can cause an inflammatory condition of the kidneys that can leave users with long-term impairment of kidney function.[2] Although it is not clear at this point why these med-

Research Can Raise More Questions than Answers

In the fall of 2007, the pharmaceutical company Astra-Zeneca—makers of Nexium and Prilosec—sent data to the FDA that, according to the agency, "raised concerns that long-term use of Prilosec or Nexium may have increased the risk of heart attacks, heart failure, and heart-related sudden death" in patients taking the drugs, compared to those who had undergone surgery instead. Stock prices dropped. The FDA spent several months reviewing data. They then concluded that there was no clear-cut association between the drugs and the diseases. However, they also acknowledged problems with the way data was collected and admitted having trouble with the analysis. As a proponent of natural remedies before medications or surgery, I wish there was a way for the agency to incorporate these methods into the study! Regardless of the study's possible shortcomings, the possible cardiovascular effects of the two popular heartburn medications do not need to be addressed in either advertising or package inserts as a result of the FDA's finding.

At the same time, advertisements for Prilosec OTC advise consumers to "[u]se as directed for fourteen days for treating frequent heartburn. Not for immediate relief." This statement baffles me. If the pill doesn't bring immediate relief, wouldn't that mean that you have to take the drug *before* the acid reflux actually occurs? I would imagine that means that after a few days, a consumer wouldn't even know if he was still having heartburn. The long-term usage that often results is simple to understand when we also consider that getting off the drug can cause rebound acid production. Where does it stop?

ications can have such a negative effect on the kidneys, it is theorized that it may be because there are proton pump receptors located within the kidneys that react when they come into contact with the PPIs.

One chemical component of Prevacid is the element fluoride. Fluoride, a toxic waste from the manufacture of aluminum, is an additive to tap water that was added in hopes of reducing dental cavities. Its critics point out that fluoride is more toxic than lead and has not been proven to improve dental health when added to drinking water. This toxin has negative effects on many body parts and systems, including bones, brain, hormones, thyroid, joints, liver, and kidneys. It may even be a carcinogen and an aging factor. Scientists at the Environmental Protection Agency, the National Academy of Sciences, the Centers for Disease Control, and many other groups are very concerned about the fluoridation of water. Several foreign countries forbid fluoride's use in water. The form in the medication is not exactly the same as the form in the water, but common sense would say to be cautious of any unnecessary long-term exposure.

Proton pump inhibitors delay the emptying of the stomach.[3] (The reasons for that will become clear as you read about the normal functioning of the digestive process.) Unfortunately, the longer the stomach contains a digestive solution, the longer you will have to be careful not to lie down or bend over so as to avoid having those fluids get into the esophagus. This is true even if the digestive fluid contains weakened acid.

The real effects of the PPIs on the gastrointestinal (GI) mucosa, especially when *H. pylori* bacterium is present, are the subject of confusing scientific discussions.[4] PPIs are routinely used as a part of the treatment for *H. pylori*, but recent animal research leads us to believe that doing so may not be necessary and may, in fact, make eradication harder.[5]

H₂-RECEPTOR ANTAGONISTS

Tagamet, Zantac, Mylanta, and Pepcid AC are members of an older class of drugs called *histamine-receptor antagonists*, or *H₂-receptor antagonists*. These medications don't stop stomach acid production as thoroughly or for as long as the PPIs. Therefore, doctors consider them less effective in easing heartburn symptoms. While they may also be somewhat safer than PPIs, these medications must still be taken with great caution. There are dozens of potential side effects from taking these drugs. Most are similar to those listed previously for PPIs. Rather than re-list them here, I am going to highlight a few particularly serious long-term side effects.

A recent study showed that elderly African Americans were two-and-a-half times more likely to have dementia if they were taking Zantac, Pepcid, or Tagamet than if they did not take one of these medications. The study did not look at Caucasians but it is believed that the findings would be similar.[6]

Tagamet has been shown to significantly increase estradiol (estrogen) in men, which can result in gynecomastia[7] (enlarged breasts) and sexual dysfunction.[8] Additionally, many experts suspect that an excess of estrogen in men may lead to prostate cancer.

Tagamet can also be dangerous when taken with the anticoagulant (blood thinner) Coumadin (warfarin). It can cause Coumadin to accumulate, which can lead to dangerous bleeding. This is particularly unfortunate because of the large number of seniors who take both Coumadin and Tagamet—which is now available without a prescription.

Antacids

These warnings regarding the newer classes of acid blockers may tempt you to go back to the older over-the-counter antacid medicines. But although these drugs may not shut down acid for such long periods of time, that doesn't mean they don't have powerful consequences. For example, one ingredient in Alka-Seltzer is aspirin. Aspirin is a non-steroidal anti-inflammatory drug (NSAID). These drugs are a leading cause of ulcers—and ulcers are a common cause of stomach pain.

Some antacids, such as Maalox, Di-Gel, and Mylanta, contain aluminum. Studies have shown that the brain matter of people with Alzheimer's disease contains a concentration of aluminum in the tangles that results in dementia. Other studies have shown that elevated aluminum in the blood is associated with a reduction in mental capacity of dialysis patients. Aluminum also interferes with the absorption of iron, so anyone prone to anemia is ill-advised to take these medications. Why not avoid aluminum sources when possible? I don't even like the idea of cooking in aluminum pots and pans—especially when I am cooking acidic foods that readily leach out the aluminum.

Tums is advertised not only as an antacid but as a source of supplemental calcium. However, the form of calcium it contains, calcium carbonate, is a cheap and not very absorbable form of the mineral. Also, the calcium in the antacid is not balanced with the other nutrients—including magnesium and Vitamin D—needed to escort that calcium through absorption and assimilation into bone. Excess calcium intake can cause constipation and is a deterrent to absorbing zinc. As a result of these factors, there are questions regarding just how helpful this supplemental calcium actually is. Excess calcium aimlessly wandering around the body has been implicated in bone spurs, kidney stones, atherosclerosis, and even prostate cancer.[9] Because calcium interferes with the uptake of thyroid medication, Tums—like other sources of calcium—shouldn't be taken within a couple of hours of taking thyroid medication.

Statistics show that people survive the *immediate* effects of these drugs. Unfortunately, all bets are off if these acid-blocking medications are taken for longer than the time for which they have been studied and are recommended—which is usually no longer than two, four, or eight weeks. The most insidious damage from these powerful medicines appears to be caused by exactly the function for which they are prescribed—reduction of stomach acid. Chapter 4 will explain why long-term interference with stomach acid production is courting health disaster.

HEARTBURN MEDICATIONS THAT DON'T BLOCK ACID

Although less common than the medications mentioned above, there are several heartburn drugs whose mode of action is not to suppress acid but rather to address heartburn in different—if not necessarily safer—ways.

One such example was the drug Propulsid. Its aim was to strengthen the esophageal sphincter and speed the movement of food through the stomach. However, this medication was removed from the market because it caused a high incidence of fatal heart arrhythmias.

Reglan (metoclopramide) is another drug for heartburn that isn't for acid suppression. It strengthens the lower esophageal sphincter (LES) and moves intestinal contents through faster. Strengthening the LES seems like a good idea, and moving food through the system faster can help—as long as the food is actually digested on its way. However, there are often unintended consequences when you force the body to do things. For example, the published side effects include uncontrollable movements of extremities, tongue, or other body part; unexplained anxiety; shortness of breath; and depression with thoughts of suicide. People taking this medicine are advised against driving a car or operating machinery. Hallucinations, although rare, are another reported side effect.

I trust you will agree that the closer we look at side effects of these pharmaceuticals, the more attractive the natural remedies sound.

IMPORTANT CONSIDERATIONS
WHEN TAKING PRESCRIPTION DRUGS

Please understand that I'm not saying that you should *never* take acid-blocking drugs. If your doctor says your esophagus is being eaten away or you have a confirmed ulcer, you might need such a drug for a very short time while you are healing. (If it is not a bleeding emergency, you may be able to heal even those problems with natural solutions.) At least consider uti-

Acid-Blocking Medications and Children

This chapter has detailed many of the short- and long-term effects that acid-blocking drugs can have on overall health. The crucial role of stomach acid, described in Chapter 4, will bring to light further reasons as to why limiting the stomach's acid production can be extremely harmful and counterproductive. I therefore find it shocking that in February of 2008 the FDA approved the use of Nexium in children ages one to eleven. More recently, I was equally surprised to see Maalox for children in a drug store. The playfully colorful packaging featured a pint-sized superhero and instructions that it can be used for children as young as two.

In my opinion, there are too many health risks for acid blockers to be a viable alternative for most children. After all, low stomach acid can cause rickets—a softening of the bones—and a host of other effects. I also consider it unwholesome to send a child the message that it is wise to take a medication rather than solving the problem.

lizing the time you are on the medicine to figure out the root cause of your pain. If you haven't changed anything else, the pain will most likely come back when you stop taking the drug, leading to a continuation of the medication. The next episode may even be worse because of rebound acid production associated with some of the medicines. Furthermore, be advised that your digestive competence is diminished while on an acid blocker. This loss can create downstream effects on nutrient storage, your ability to make proper digestive juices, and your ability to continue healing damage. Following are some important factors to keep in mind, not only with acid-blockers but *any* prescription medication.

• Drugs must be patented to be profitable. To achieve a patentable product, the pharmaceutical companies create a molecule that has never been on the planet before. Therefore, most drugs are, by definition, foreign to the body. The body has not learned to cope with the chemical and you can't blame nature if something goes wrong.

• Virtually all drugs have side effects. Other than immunizations and a few of what I call "replacers" (such as insulin and thyroid hormone), most drugs are "anti"-this (such as anti-inflammatory) or "antagonist" that (such as histamine-receptor antagonists) or "so-and-so" blocker (calcium channel blockers). This is because most drugs are created as poisons programmed to interfere with one of the body's chemical pathways or systems to take the load off another one that is producing the undesirable symptoms. Unfortunately, there is always a price to pay when you block a pathway that also performs some good functions. The same is true for drugs that speed up a process against the body's inclination. Lipitor, one of the statin drugs dispensed for lowering cholesterol, is one such example. It is designed to inhibit an enzyme involved in the production of cholesterol. Yet Lipitor also blocks the pathway that makes coenzyme Q_{10}. This enzyme is responsible for creating most of the cellular energy in the body. Lipitor, therefore, reduces the body's ability to make CoQ_{10}, causing many of the reported side effects.

Non-steroidal anti-inflammatory drugs (NSAIDs) are another example of a blocker. They keep the body from generating its natural response—inflammation—to an irritant of some kind. As a result, pain is reduced, but in the process, the drug may also keep the body from repairing the damaged organ. NSAIDs affect the liver, kidneys, and heart, and can cause ulcers and death. That 16,500 people in the United States die each year from this one class of drugs should be a serious wakeup call. (I suggest reading *Pain Free in 6 Weeks* by Sherry Rogers, MD, for safer solutions to joint pain.)

• Most drugs are designed only to alleviate a symptom, not solve the problem that caused the symptom. The underlying issue may continue to get worse and because your alarm system (the symptom) has been turned off, you are unaware that your health is still suffering.

• Some drugs can ultimately worsen the underlying cause of the condition they were supposed to address. That leads to greater usage over time. Dr. Rogers says this is one way "the sick get sicker quicker." In this book, you are going to read in detail how that principle works with heartburn drugs.

• Each person has a different level of susceptibility to each side effect. Some people detoxify poorly, which allows drugs to build up to higher than expected levels in their systems. Some process drugs too quickly to achieve the desired effect. Genetic makeup and age are both factors. Even gender makes a difference. Until recently, most drug testing was done only on men. Now, however, we know that women tend to detoxify drugs slower than men. Regardless, you must carefully monitor everything that changes when you take a drug because the statistics on dosage and side effects do not necessarily apply to you—because you are a unique individual, not a statistic.

Environment can also change how drugs are handled. For example, if you are exposed to toxins in your work environment or live in a new mobile home that is off-gassing formaldehyde, your detoxification pathways may already be too busy dealing with your environment to deal with the medication.

• You could be allergic to the medicine. Signs of an allergic reaction can include swelling of face or tongue, trouble swallowing, asthma-like wheezing, or loss of consciousness. Less serious signs of a reaction might be anything from red ears to hives.

• Side effects may not be noticed right away. If you pass out an hour after you take a medication, you will most likely attribute the problem to the drug. However, if you experience muscle wasting months or even years after you begin taking a cholesterol-lowering medicine, it is possible that you nor your doctor will think to associate that condition with the drug.

At the same time, initial research may not be asking the right questions. The Merck drug Vioxx was hailed as an NSAID with less gastrointestinal risk, which is the effect the company was looking for. However, it was recalled in 2004 because it significantly increased the risk of heart attacks and strokes. Later studies aimed at Alzheimer's prevention showed that the drug also *tripled* deaths from all causes among those patients.

• Side effects usually have the potential to be more dangerous if label instructions aren't followed. Accidental overdose is the most obvious of these problems. Sometimes that happens because an elderly person forgets they already took their medicine. If this occurs, call 911, your doctor, or poison control center, or go straight to the emergency room. A more subtle way than overdose to foil the safety limits in the prescription instructions is to continuously take a drug that was intended only for short-term use. As I mentioned, virtually all acid-blocking drugs have only been approved for temporary use of a few weeks.

• You must read the package insert. Yes, the print is exceedingly small and the language intimidating. However, the warnings change as new information is discovered, so please read this print every time your prescription is refilled or you pick up another over-the-counter medication.

• Stopping abruptly can be dangerous. With some drugs (such as psychiatric medications), going off cold turkey can be life threatening. Acid blockers should be tapered off to avoid rebound acid production.

• The effect of your medication can either increase or decrease depending on the substances—usually drugs, food, or beverages—with which it interacts. For example, Nexium keeps some antibiotics from working properly. Also, acid blockers prescribed along with non-steroidal anti-inflammatory drugs (NSAIDs) can cause ulcers, especially among seniors. There are many other combinations of which you and your doctor must be aware.

Medication can also react with some foods. For example, if a person takes the cholesterol-lowering medication Lovastatin and drinks grapefruit juice, the levels of the drug can build up dramatically (as much as twelve times the normal levels, according to one study).[10] This effect can last for twenty-four hours. Some doctors tell their patients who are taking Coumadin (warfarin) to avoid broccoli, cabbage, and Brussels sprouts because they contain vitamin K, which may decrease the effectiveness of the drug. However, these are all healthy, cancer-fighting foods. Other doctors wisely advise patients to keep their intake of those nutritious foods relatively constant and adjust the dose of the drug around them.

Many medications can be extremely dangerous when combined with alcohol. Tylenol (acetaminophen), for example, can combine with alcohol to create fatal liver damage.

Just because a product is available without a prescription does not mean it is necessarily safe. You must be aware of the effects of all the herbs and dietary supplements you take and their effects when combined with medications. The herb St. John's Wort, which is effective for moderate depression, detoxifies some drugs and lessens their effects. That means that someone who had an organ transplant and is on anti-rejection medication should avoid this herb. Personally, I have found that the antioxidant vitamin C, when taken before a trip to the dentist, causes the anesthetic to detoxify before I'm ready for it to leave my system. Enteric-coated peppermint oil is beneficial for irritable bowel but can cause heartburn in a susceptible person.

• Just as nutrients may interfere with your medicine, prescription drugs often interfere with your nutrients. Virtually every prescription comes with documentation that states which nutrients may suffer as a result of taking the drug. The medicine can interfere with uptake of the nutrient (such as what acid blockers do with minerals), it can block some conversion required for utilization, or your body may draft some of your stored nutrients in an attempt to make the drug less toxic and/or get rid of it.

• Always evaluate both the risks and the benefits of every medication you take. The FDA approves drugs despite risks if it feels that the benefits outweigh the risks. Drugs are removed from the market when the risk/benefit equation no longer makes sense. Ultimately, it is up to you to decide if the benefit you receive is worth the price you may pay. For example, once you know safer natural alternatives to the acid blockers, you may decide that risking dementia, heart disease, pneumonia, liver failure, osteoporosis, and cancer is too high a price for relieving acid indigestion through prescribed medication.

• Cost is a consideration. Medicines are expensive. Additionally, their cost is an expense that goes on forever if the underlying problem isn't solved. Those with good insurance often become complacent about the financial aspect, but that is a shortsighted view. There may not be a guarantee that the insurance coverage will continue. Also, the costs trickle down and reappear in taxes and the cost of goods and services. Don't forget that the biggest cost may be in the gradual deterioration of your health.

• As a consumer, you must always remember that drug companies are part of a savvy profit-driven industry. Their accountability is, in large part, to their shareholders rather than the public. Collectively, these companies spend almost $5 billion in annual drug advertising; as consumers, we should not allow this bombardment of ads to influence our decisions.

Although we hope that the US Food and Drug Administration is adequately protecting the medications that hit the shelves of our pharmacies, it is overworked and underfunded. At the same time, some studies also show that the drug companies exert worrisome influence over medical schools, state groups that set practice standards, the media, and even lawmakers. In fact, there are more than twice as many pharmaceutical lobbyists as there are lawmakers in Washington, DC. It is clear that we need to stay informed in order to make the best decisions for the health of ourselves and our families.

NON-DRUG CONVENTIONAL APPROACH

Drugs are not the only mainstream treatment for heartburn. Conventional medicine also offers a surgical option. This surgery shares the risks common to all surgery, up to and including death. (I have heard it said that the only "minor surgery" is one that someone else is having.) *Consumer Reports* said, "Research shows the operation, which costs $14,600 or more, provides no better long-term relief than taking a proton-pump inhibitor drug." The surgery may also damage digestion over the long haul. After considering both medications and surgery, my opinion is that it is only logical that the first attempt to solve the pain of heartburn should be with natural means.

RIGHT ANSWER TO THE WRONG QUESTION

In my opinion, we will one day look back and view many of these medical interventions as nearly barbaric. Regardless of whether the misguided advice from the medical community has been well intended, consumers have been led to believe they should find a way to stop the production of stomach acid. In reality, the question consumers should ask is what non-toxic actions they can take to allow acid to continue doing its job without allowing it to travel outside the areas it is supposed to be. The need for stomach acid will become clearer in the next chapter, which discusses its role and benefits.

CHAPTER 4

STOMACH ACID:
A CURSE OR A BLESSING?

*"It is more important to know what sort of person
has a disease than to know what sort of disease a person has."*
—HIPPOCRATES

Hippocrates, credited with being the father of medicine, wasn't distracted by the glitter of today's high-tech medical machinery and medications. He practiced around 300 BC in Greece, and his most critical tools were careful observation and the ability to think things through. My guess is that he would find it illogical to give a person drugs to entirely stop stomach acid production without first determining if too much acid is the problem. Maybe we need to bring back his practical way of thinking.

Hyperchlorhydria is a relatively rare condition in which the body produces excess digestive juice, including stomach acid. This condition is most often called Zollinger-Ellison syndrome, which involves tumors in the pancreas or small intestine. The overproduction of fluids may then result in duodenal (small intestine) ulcers.

However, most people who are prescribed acid blockers are actually suffering from *low* stomach acid. This is a common condition called *hypochlorhydria*. In *Why Stomach Acid Is Good for You*, renowned nutrition-oriented physician Jonathan Wright, MD, notes, "I've observed that nine out of ten of us who suffer from so-called 'acid indigestion' actually have *lack-*

of-acid indigestion." Other estimates are lower, claiming that closer to half of sufferers have too little acid. Either way, the insufficiency affects lot of people. Yet mainstream medicine balks at even entertaining the idea that a fundamental cause of heartburn and GERD might be that meals and weak acid are staying in the stomach too long because the acid is simply not concentrated enough to do the required digestion. The stomach contents can then brew and bubble, slosh around for an extended period, and enter the delicate esophagus. Another danger of low acidity in the stomach, whether pre-existing or drug-induced, is that the environment may not be sufficiently sterile to keep bacteria from setting up shop and damaging the stomach lining. Inadequate digestion can also result in poor nutrient absorption, which in turn hampers repair of the damage. And so the cycle begins.

Most of the problems for which acid blockers are prescribed are due to the contact of acid with tissues that are not properly protected from it. This is usually because either the acid has traveled to a body part, such as the esophagus, where it does not belong, or the acid is in contact with stomach or intestinal tissues that are in a poor state of repair and have bare spots in the normal protective mucous layer.

To better understand not only what is happening but why taking acid blockers for extended periods of time may actually worsen the problem, let's first take a look at the important role of stomach acid in digestion.

WHAT IS GASTRIC JUICE?

The body has an elegant system for prioritizing its use of materials and energy. It uses a lot of its resources to make roughly two quarts of stomach acid every day. Stomach acid, which is also called gastric acid, is commonly thought to be solely hydrochloric acid (HCl), but it also contains other materials.

Among the constituents are water, electrolyte minerals (potassium, chloride, and sodium chloride), enzymes, intrinsic factor (which is required for the absorption of vitamin B_{12}), and a little mucus. The solution should be very, very acidic. On a pH scale of -1 to +14 (where -1 is the most acidic and 14 the most alkaline), stomach HCl hovers at the extreme low end, varying from 1 to 3. (For comparison, consider that full-strength acid in your car battery has a pH of slightly less than 1.) HCl is secreted by special cells in the stomach called parietal cells.

THE IMPORTANCE OF GASTRIC ACID

Food is not absorbed in the stomach (although alcohol is) but what happens there is crucial to the rest of the digestive process. As you will read, there are many reasons for this.

The Role of Gastric Acid in Digestion

The stomach is programmed to empty at a certain stage of digestion. Gastric acid is crucial to the process of digestion and ensuring it occurs at the proper speed. If the strength of the acid is too low, the stomach step of digestion doesn't get completed and the food hangs around. The continued presence of food in the stomach generates the perceived need for more acid. The body then responds to the call and more fluid might build up, but it will probably be equally weak and ineffective. While the mixture lingers in the warmth of the stomach, carbohydrates in the meal can ferment, creating alcohol and gas bubbles. If splashed into the esophagus, even a weak acid or acid/alcohol mixture will burn the tissues found there because they are not designed to be acid resistant.

In addition to its roles in the stomach, gastric acid triggers a chain reaction of other processes up and down the line in the digestive tract. The body has untold numbers of signaling mechanisms, called "feedback loops." One of the messages sent by stomach acid is that the lower esophageal sphincter (LES) should close. If the stomach acid content is low, that signal may not function properly. Another feedback miscue, as Allan Spreen, MD, points out, is that when the HCl is continuously low, the body may not work as hard to protect the esophagus. Its energy and materials will be routed to a body part perceived to be in greater need.

Without the presence of HCl, protein digestion cannot begin. Stomach acid first unfolds proteins in the food and then activates another digestive substance—pepsin—which breaks down the proteins into smaller units called peptides. Then, enzymes in the small intestines further break down these peptides into amino acids. Stomach acid signals for the release of these enzymes. If stomach acid has been blocked or becomes insufficient, much of the protein may not release its amino acids and instead will rot.

Amino acids are extremely important to health and function. They are commonly known as the building blocks of muscle, but they are also required to build body parts including the kidney, liver, blood, bone, skin, and hair. Amino acids are also part of hormones, enzymes, neurotransmitters, and other signaling chemicals. They are needed to repair damaged esophageal tissues and to strengthen the LES muscle if it has become weakened. Therefore, since gastric acid is required to produce sufficient amounts of amino acids, low acid may well mean low esophageal repair and low LES strength. If eso-phageal tissues are not sufficiently repaired, they can be further irritated by even the weakly acidic stomach contents that leak into the esophagus through a weakened valve. This often leads sufferers to take more acid blockers—resulting in a vicious cycle.

Stomach acid also sends a signal down the line that tells the next stage of digestion to prepare bicarbonate, which neutralizes the acid coming out of the stomach. The upper part of the small intestine, in which most digestive enzymes operate, must be alkaline for the enzymes to function. When there is less acid in the stomach, the body releases less bicarbonate and the proper alkalinity isn't achieved. That in turn affects the release and effect of enzymes that should process and prepare various food components for breakdown and absorption. So, in short, low stomach acid breaks the digestive chain.

Gastric Acid as Our First Line of Defense

Stomach acid is our first line of defense against invading bacteria, fungus, parasites, viruses, and allergic substances. Even airborne allergens that go in through the nose end up in the stomach. If we short circuit that line of defense by lowering stomach acid, pathogens like bacteria have easy access. This can lead to an imbalance of helpful versus harmful bacteria in the intestinal tract. The imbalance can, in turn, cause a breakdown of the intestinal barrier, which may foster autoimmune conditions. Not all of the potential disease connections have been researched, but studies do show that low acid creates an increased risk of dying of pneumonia. Insufficient acid increases the risk of infection with the dangerous diarrhea-producing *C. difficile* bacterium and food poisoning from *E. coli* or salmonella bugs. *H. pylori* (a cause of gastritis and ulcers), too, is thought to usually first occur when the level of acid in the stomach is low.

Gastric Acid and the Absorption of Nutrients

One of the many functions of gastric acid is to assist your digestion with the absorption of nutrients. There are vitamins and minerals that cannot be adequately absorbed without the help of this fluid. Therefore, most people with low levels of stomach acidity have a reduced ability to absorb the nutrients they need.

Vitamin Absorption

Stomach acid is required for the chain of events that allows for the absorption of vitamin B_{12}. Inadequate B_{12} can cause many serious problems, including short-term memory loss, permanent damage to the nervous system, depressed moods, confusion, loss of mental sharpness, constipation, numbness in extremities, loss of strength in the arms and legs, and, new research suggests, rectal cancer. Low levels of this vitamin also reduce energy levels. Many people feel less fatigued after a shot of B_{12}. Although I have not seen any research on the subject, I theorize that low B_{12} levels may also weaken the LES! Unfortunately, B_{12} levels are also already under attack by a number of other drugs in addition to acid blockers, such as metformin, an anti-diabetic drug.

Low stomach acid also interrupts a normal chain reaction that results in the absorption of another important B vitamin: folic acid. Folic acid is plentiful in green vegetables but is destroyed by cooking. Fat metabolism, the creation and repair of our genetic code, the health of our arteries, and the health of our brain all depend on folic acid. The prevention of spina bifida (a neural tube birth defect) is among the benefits of folic acid. Research published in 2007 showed that post-menopausal women who consumed the greatest amount of folate had a 44-percent lower risk of breast cancer than those who consumed the least.[1] A Swedish study linked folic acid to reducing the risk of ovarian cancer, especially among women who consume alcohol.[2] Folic acid works with vitamins B_{12} and B_6 to lower homocysteine, a toxic amino acid in the blood that is a potent cancer, heart attack, and stroke risk factor.[3] Like vitamin B_{12}, B_6 and folic acid are already routinely reduced by many factors, including birth control pills and other medicines.

Mineral Absorption

There is a general assumption in the medical community that acid-suppressing medicines do not interfere with mineral absorption. A couple of short-duration studies seem to support that view. However, the longer-term studies and the growing list of acid-blocker side effects may be telling a different story. Gastric acid certainly assists in the absorption of certain essential minerals, so it stands to reason that decreasing the acid may slow this process.

Nutrition textbooks have long held that acid is important in the absorption of magnesium. This mineral keeps the heart beating properly. It is also an anti-inflammatory and is needed to protect the arteries from arteriosclerosis, clots, and high blood pressure.[4] Magnesium's relationship to glucose uptake might be an important factor in metabolic syndrome and could be the missing link between type II diabetes and high blood pressure.[5, 6] Magnesium has many, many more important roles, including working to prevent asthma, anxiety, depression, muscle spasms, osteoporosis, gallstones, and constipation. Magnesium sufficiency has even been linked to reduced risk of lung cancer and shown to decrease risk of metastasis in cancer patients.[7] Unfortunately, magnesium is deficient in the commercial food supply and is systematically eliminated in food processing. A whopping 70 percent of the population consumes less than the modest recommended daily intake.[8] On top of that, many drugs, including anti-inflammatories, some antibiotics, birth control pills, Digoxin, and diuretics, further deplete the body of magnesium. Hypochlorhydria only worsens this problem by decreasing the body's ability to absorb this important mineral.

Acid is required to absorb zinc, another mineral already in widespread deficiency.[9, 10] Zinc is leached from the soil of most farmland and since it is not required for all crops, there is no economic incentive to add it to all fertilizers. Yet zinc is used in some 120 extremely important enzyme systems in the body. It is needed, for instance, for the thyroid to work properly. Zinc helps prevent insulin resistance, cataracts, and blindness from macular degeneration.[11] It is also involved in building bone and maintaining cell membranes and hormone balance. Zinc is crucial for healing tissues—including those that may need restoration in the esophagus and stomach. It is important to proper function of the immune system, which protects us from infectious disease and cancer. It has been shown to be particularly preventive against esophageal cancer.[12] Therefore, when we lower stomach acid with acid-blocking drugs and interfere with zinc uptake, we increase the chance of developing a cancer in the very tissues that the medication was taken to protect. Deficiencies of zinc, selenium, and other nutrients affected by stomach acid are linked to macular degeneration, a serious condition that limits sight, particularly in the elderly. The appearance of white spots on the fingernails is one sign of zinc deficiency. In the short term, the drugs may relieve pain and offer some protection while tissues heal. However, you can see how long-term use of these medications can undermine the repair process and ensure that the need for the acid blockers will never end.

Gastric acid is used in the absorption of calcium, particularly when consumed in supplements. It works to separate the calcium from whatever it is bound to. Calcium has an untold number of roles in our chemistry, from transmitting nerve impulses to helping muscles work. (It is worth noting that the LES—as well as the heart—is a muscle.) Additionally, although the exact mechanism isn't known, studies have shown that long-term use of acid blockers increases the risk of hip fracture. As American consumers, we've had it drilled into us by various economic interests and some well-meaning authorities that calcium is needed to build strong bones. While there is truth to that claim, we have gotten carried away, consuming more calcium than any population on the planet. Yet we also hold the record for the highest rate of osteoporosis. We have been blindly concentrating on calcium to the exclusion of the other nutrients needed to build bone. These include magnesium and zinc.[13]

There are shockingly few studies on the relationship between acid blockers and mineral absorption. The few that do exist conflict. In 1996, Tufts University did a spot check of eight people after one meal and concluded there was no problem with short-term use of PPIs.[14] Since that time, evidence (such as the increase in risk of hip fractures) has started to accumulate, suggesting that mineral metabolism is upset by acid-blocking medication.

Gastric Acid's Effect on the Thyroid

The thyroid gland is crucial for health. When it is under functioning, it can produce many negative effects, including reduced immune function, depression, dry skin, thinning hair, constipation, increased cholesterol, and fatigue. It also adversely affects the rate of metabolism within the body and can lead to weight gain. The thyroid gland requires zinc and magnesium, as well as vitamin A, B-complex vitamins, iodine, selenium, fatty acids, and the amino acid tyrosine, to function properly. These nutrients depend on stomach acid to start the digestive process that fosters their absorption. Acid-blocking drugs, therefore, are likely to decrease the absorption of the important nutrients that affect the efficiency of the thyroid gland. At the same time, thyroid medications such as levothyroxine are not well absorbed by people with low stomach acid, according to a 2006 study. We can begin to see how we can inadvertently turn a delicate balance into a vicious downward spiral if we remove a key natural element of digestion such as stomach acid. There are other indirect connections and probably many yet to be discovered.

Gastric Acid and Depression

Stomach acid helps avoid depression in several ways. The depletion of neurotransmitters, particularly serotonin, is often heavily involved in depression, and stomach acid helps break down protein into amino acids, which are then made into neurotransmitters. Another requirement for the formation of neurotransmitters is vitamin B_{12} and, as discussed on page 48, the absorption of this vitamin requires acid. The bulk of serotonin production and receptors are in the intestinal tract, and stomach acid is indirectly involved in keeping that department healthy. Low acid can also contribute to overgrowth of intestinal yeast that is associated with depression. Magnesium deficiency is related to depression, and there is a connection between stomach acid and magnesium absorption, as you read on page 49. Is it any wonder that depression is listed as a potential side effect of proton pump inhibitors? At the same time, many people who take the popular anti-depressant Prozac report that it gives them heartburn—which certainly seems the beginning of a vicious cyle.

Other Connections to Gastric Acid

When gastric acid is low, there is no guarantee that the body will be able to adequately absorb important fatty acids and fat-soluble vitamins. This is because insufficient acid can result in only partial digestion. Also, the meal remnants remain in the GI tract and break down into toxic elements that can be absorbed and cause a myriad of problems. Deficiencies in zinc and calcium can allow more toxic metals such as cadmium and aluminum to collect. This toxicity can disrupt many normal body processes.

Because vegetarians don't eat red meat, they are at risk of getting too little iron and zinc from their diets. As a result, they are much more dependent on stomach acid to pull minerals from plant sources, particularly those in which the minerals are tightly bound until released by digestive juices. Vegetarians are also more prone to B_{12} deficiencies. Therefore, vegetarians must be especially careful not to tamper with stomach acid.

Stomach acid helps prevent gallbladder disease because of its role in the chain reaction that stimulates the flow of bile. Without stomach acid, on the other hand, bile can concentrate in the gallbladder and cause stones to precipitate. (You already read about the connection between stomach acid and magnesium, a mineral that is protective against gallstones.)

DO YOU HAVE LOW GASTRIC ACID?

You have read about the many health conditions associated with low stomach acid. If you are taking an acid-suppressing medication, your stomach acid is probably insufficient. It may, however, be low even if you are not taking an acid blocker. This section will take a look at the signs that may point to a deficiency in your gastric acid. It also offers ways to replenish the deficiency.

Evaluating Your Stomach Acid

When a person has low stomach acid, there are many different factors that can affect how his or her symptoms appear. These include age, genetics, habits, diet, environment, and the length of time the acid has been low. Therefore, and because stomach acid has many primary and indirect uses, the clues to acid insufficiency are surprisingly many and diverse. Sufferers may exhibit only one of the following signs, or they may exhibit several. Any one of these conditions can be caused by or compounded by other factors besides low acid. Generally, however, the more clues you exhibit, the more likely that you are in need of more or stronger stomach acid. If you experienced one of these problems in the past but it is now being controlled by medication, it should still be counted.

Some of the conditions on the following list may in fact be causes of as well as symptoms of low stomach acid. Here, we face the problem of the chicken or the egg. Let's consider a Candida yeast infection as an example. The low stomach acid may have initially allowed the yeast to settle in. The yeast condition then worsens the low stomach acid because of its actions in the gut. The low acid fosters the continuation of the yeast condition. Yeast infections will be further discussed in Chapter 6, but you can see the difficulty in determining whether certain conditions are cause or effect.

Any of the following conditions may appear along with low stomach acid:

- Addison's disease (severely underfunctioning adrenal glands)

- Anemia or an iron deficiency

- Asthma

- Autoimmune disease (such as chronic autoimmune hepatitis, Graves' disease, lupus, multiple sclerosis, myasthenia gravis, polymyalgia rheumatica, Reynaud's syndrome, rheumatoid arthritis, scleroderma, Sjögren's syndrome, type I diabetes, and vitiligo—spotty loss of skin pigment)

- Bacterial overgrowth in the gut

- Belching

- Bloating

- Candida yeast infection

- Celiac/sprue
- Constipation
- Diarrhea
- Fatigue
- Feeling that food just sits in the stomach
- Food sensitivities
- Foul breath and/or gas
- Gallbladder disease
- Hair that is thin, weak, or brittle
- Heartburn/acid reflux after meals
- Hungry all the time
- Inability to eat large meals
- Longitudinal ridges in your fingernails, weak/brittle nails
- Loss of appetite for meat
- Macular degeneration
- Nausea after taking supplements
- Osteoporosis or osteopenia
- Skin issues such as acne rosacea, psoriasis, eczema, or dilated capillaries on the face
- Thin, fragile, dry skin
- Ulcerative colitis

Testing Your Stomach Acid

The clues in the previous section may have given you an indication that your acid levels are too low. If so, there are several available lab tests that can confirm or reject this suspicion.

The Heidelberg Gastric Analysis test is very accurate, but also expensive and very hard to find. The doctor gives the patient a radio-transmitting capsule to swallow. The capsule transmits information regarding the stomach's pH level, which is then plotted on a graph. The pill later passes through with the waste.

The "Gastro-Test" is less expensive than the Heidelberg Gastric Analysis test. It is also somewhat less accurate. In this test, a capsule connected to a string is swallowed while one end of the string is held outside the body. The capsule then sits in the stomach long enough to dissolve and expose the string to the gastric juice. At that point, the string is pulled out. Its color indicates the stomach's pH. This test can also be used as a check for GERD, so be sure the doctor understands you want to test your *stomach* pH, not just that of your esophagus.

A third test for the acidity of gastric acid is a blood test called the blood quininium resin test (bQRT). Research indicates that this test is accurate. Unfortunately, it is not yet widely available. Hopefully, as respect for our need for stomach acid increases, this test will become commercially viable.[15]

Some people employ another option: trial and error. Rather than using any of the above tests, they check the sufficiency of their stomach acid by treating the situation as though their stomach acid is, in fact, low. If one of the acid-boosting remedies they try leads to an improvement in the problem, their stomach acid was most likely low.

Improving Your Stomach Acid

It is rare to get information from an HMO about increasing stomach acid. That is because the conventional system is to suppress the symptom. A PPI is a quick fix and suits its business model better than the more difficult work of determining the underlying cause of the heartburn. Therefore, most of the information regarding improving your level of stomach acid is from the advice of the respected experts in the field of natural medicine who routinely and effectively treat heartburn patients without the use of acid-blocking drugs.

Address the Root Cause

If your stomach acid is low, the most logical and effective route is to curtail whatever caused it to be low in the first place. The method may, of course, depend on the problem. Regardless of the situation, you must stop taking acid-blocking or -absorbing medications if you need more stomach acid. Antacids will neutralize what little acid you have. They also push blood to become more alkaline, which reduces the body's ability to create more stomach acid.

Another relatively easy yet effective way to avoid interfering with acid production is to steer clear of tap water that contains chlorine and fluoride. Dr. Wright says that these minerals lower the amount of enzymes that help the stomach make acid. (Please note that most water filtration systems do not remove fluoride from tap water. See the Resources for one that does.) Water is important to your general health as well as your production of stomach acid and digestion, so continue to drink water—but try to stick to pure water. Also, drink mostly between meals so as not to dilute your acid.

Infection with the bacteria *H. pylori* is one potential cause of reduced stomach acid. In Chapter 6, I cover reasons for and methods of getting rid of this strain of bacteria. Overgrowth of yeast can also be a factor in reducing acid production. Chronic stress (resulting in adrenal fatigue) and excess alcohol consumption are additional reasons the acid production might be sub par. Reducing the impediments to your acid production is an effective way to deal with the problem—and has other health benefits as well.

Reduce Demand

You can also reduce the workload of your gastric acid so that the amount you have will go further and work more effectively. This can be done with better food choices (discussed in Chapter 9), by chewing more thoroughly, and with the use of plant-based enzymes (which we'll explore in Chapter 5). If you tend to eat a lot of protein and heavy foods, you may want to introduce more plant and raw foods into your diet. Supplementing with minerals that have already been acidified, such as Albion-chelated minerals, allows them to be absorbed without further taxing the acid.

Encourage Production

You can boost production of stomach acid by supplying what is needed for its manufacture and with indirect coaxing. You have little to lose by starting with these indirect methods of supporting stomach acid to see if your symptoms are alleviated. If your tissues are severely eroded, however, you may have to wait to try these until the doctor confirms that you have healed sufficiently.

A chronic underproduction of HCL could be an indication of a thiamine (B_1) or zinc deficiency. Supplementation of the appropriate nutrient may treat your problem. Some literature theorizes that vitamin D—the vitamin found in sunshine—is required for the body to form stomach acid. Is your problem worse in the winter? This could indicate your body's need for more vitamin D. Supplementing this vitamin while also eliminating some heavy foods can support your production of gastric acid.

Another low-tech method of stimulating stomach acid is the use of vinegar. Mix one teaspoon of vinegar with a small amount of water. Drink this mixture at each meal. If it burns, immediately neutralize the vinegar with a teaspoon of baking soda mixed with water. If the vinegar is tolerated, on the other hand, you can gradually increase the amount until you are taking six teaspoons of vinegar (diluted in water) with each meal. Unrefined Bragg organic apple cider vinegar is a good choice. You can also use lemon juice instead of vinegar.

You may recall that gastric acid is composed in large part of hydrochloric acid. There is, of course, a chloride component to this solution. After the acid is produced, the stomach releases sodium bicarbonate into blood circulation. The sodium is then used to make acid-buffering sodium bicarbonate in the small intestine. Without this, the pancreatic enzymes wouldn't work. Because of these factors, I hypothesize that there may be negative effects from diets that make extreme restrictions in sodium chloride—salt. Although I could not find any studies suggesting one way or the other, there may in fact be a connection between low sodium intake and low stomach acid. On the other hand, be careful not to consume too much salt, because excess sodium causes some people to experience an increase in blood pressure. For use in cooking, I recommend the flavorful RealSalt brand because it is a natural source of unprocessed salt and contains many desirable minerals.

A time-honored and indirect way to stimulate your stomach's production of acid is with *bitters*—infusions made from herbs, fruits, and roots. Herbal bitters, such as the traditional Swedish bitters, have been used for hundreds of years as a way to improve digestion. At least in part, this effect occurs because bitters increase the amount of acid in the stomach. At the same time, they may also improve the function of the LES. Predictably, bitters taste rather bitter. The physical reaction you have to tasting it seems to be important to the effect, so do not dilute it or mask the flavor with other substances. Take bitters about four to five minutes before a meal. (They even help the flow of bile, a later digestive function that is important for the proper digestion of fatty acids and fat-soluble vitamins.) The addition of garnish, such as endive and parsley, on plates at some restaurants is often thought to be mere decoration. However, it is likely that this practice may have started because these are bitter plants and their consumption assists digestion.

Supplement with the Real Thing

Dr. Wright says the practices described in the section "Encourage Production" are not as helpful for promoting nutrient absorption as taking real hydrochloric acid in the form of betaine HCl. However, taking HCl as a supplement requires some caution. Ideally, you should have a knowledgeable health professional analyze your situation to make sure you need the supplemental acid and supervise your trial. HCl is intended for use in a stomach that has intact mucous membranes. Definitely do not take HCl if you have an ulcer. You should also not take HCl if you are taking cortisone or an NSAID (anti-inflammatory drug) because these medications may have already damaged the lining of your stomach.

Your health professional can help you determine appropriate dosage. As a frame of reference, Dr. Wright recommends 650-milligram tablets or capsules of betaine. (Some people, particularly those who have an especially hard time with protein foods, will do better with a supplement that also contains pepsin.) Many say to begin by taking one pill per meal, at the beginning of the meal, and then, if you don't react negatively to the supplement, gradually increase this dose after two or three days. Adults may require as many as five to seven capsules per meal, depending on the size of the meal. As per the advice of Dr. Allan Spreen, divide the dose if you are taking a number of these pills by taking two in the middle of the meal. Don't chew HCl pills or put them into food or beverages because it is hard on tooth enamel. If you encounter pain when taking the supplement, Dr. Liz Lipski suggests to immediately ingest one teaspoon of baking soda diluted in water. I believe that pain when taking HCl is a sign that you either have raw tissue or, less likely, did not need the acid.

In my experience, most people have enjoyed relief implementing the combination of a change in diet and habits along with consumption of a digestion enzyme that contains HCl. (The enzyme part of the equation is really important and will be discussed in the next chapter.) Therefore, I would suggest beginning with this combination product. If you and your doctor then determine you need a higher dosage of HCl, try a separate HCl supplement. As your body/stomach regains the ability to make its own acid, watch for the need to reduce the dosage. If you experience abdominal pain, burning, or dark stools, immediately discontinue the HCl supplementation.

The ideal goal is to allow your body to again make sufficient acid and repair your tissues without acid supplements. Some experts say you should hesitate to supplement HCl over the long term because you can force your blood to tap into your body's mineral reserves to buffer the resulting acidity.

Undo the Damage

If your acid has been insufficient for a long time, you might need to work a little harder at replenishing whatever has been depleted. For example, a bone scan can determine whether your bone density is normal. If it isn't, playing catch up on bone nutrients such as calcium, magnesium, manganese, boron, and vitamins D and K may be required. A broad spectrum bone supplement, such as BoneUp by Jarrow, should contain all of these. Your doctor can also test your vitamin B_{12} level. If the level is low, I'd recommend using a methylcobalamin (B_{12}) supplement that is sublingual (designed to be dissolved under the tongue) because that doesn't depend on a healthy stomach lining for absorption. I suggest the product No Shot, which is listed in the Resources. Besides working to reinvigorate the production of stomach acid, you may need to restore balance to other areas that were affected. You will find health tips throughout the following chapters that address issues such as depression, immune problems, and thyroid deficiency.

CONCLUSION

As you now can better appreciate, our body relies on stomach acid for many critical functions. Because of this, low stomach acid often results in a wide variety of symptoms. Although there are effective ways to rectify the condition, acid-blocking medications are certainly not a solution to problems created by low stomach acid. An insufficiency of enzymes is another cause of digestive distress that is not alleviated by acid-blocking drugs. The next chapter will focus on this related situation.

CHAPTER 5

DIGEST THIS, ENZYMES!

*"Life would be infinitely happier if we could only be born
at the age of eighty and gradually approach eighteen."*
—MARK TWAIN

As we get older, some of our bodily processes tend to become less effective. This is an unfortunate fact of life. However, we do have some control because the greatest part of this decline is caused by the accumulation of toxic insults and sins of nutritional omission. Prevention is the best way to reduce this damage, but, to a certain extent, existing damage can also be reversed.

Chapter 4 explained the possible effects of stomach acid insufficiency. Yet this is not the only shortcoming faced by our digestive processes. A great many Americans, particularly older folks, do not properly digest their meals because they have insufficient digestive enzymes. The situation is similar to what we see when a person has low stomach acid. Insufficient digestive enzymes can cause the incompletely digested food to hang around, causing heartburn and other short-term distress. Long-term effects of inadequate nutrition and toxicity can also result.

This chapter will begin with a basic explanation of enzymes and their role in your health. I will then offer suggestions on how to replenish deficient enzymes in an effort to alleviate your digestive troubles.

ENZYMES

At their most basic level, *enzymes* are protein substances that act as catalysts. *Catalysts* are substances that cause a chemical reaction to occur or speed up without actually participating in that reaction. Industrial enzymes are used in film processing and a host of commercial applications (such as stain removal). In humans, enzymes work all over the body, not just in the digestive tract. Each enzyme performs just one unique function, so there are thousands (perhaps hundreds of thousands) of enzymes required to keep us functioning normally. Since they are proteins, enzymes are made of amino acids, but they also require vitamins and minerals as cofactors to accomplish their jobs. If we are undernourished in any proteins or micronutrients, the effectiveness of the enzymes may be limited. Temperature and acid/alkaline balance also affect how well enzymes work.

The fact that our chemistry is largely enzyme driven provides the basis for many drugs. Some drugs suppress a symptom (in other words, stop an action in the body) by inhibiting the enzyme that is supposed to direct the related process. For example, the proton pump inhibitor class of acid blockers (which includes Nexium, Prilosec, and Prevacid) act by blocking the enzyme system known as the gastric proton pump. That system is what directs cells in the stomach to make acid. The proton pump is the last step in gastric acid secretion. The body cannot create a shortcut to make acid, so these medications effectively inhibit the acid's production. Similarly, some poisons cause harm by inhibiting an enzyme.

Metabolic Enzymes

There are two major types of enzymes: metabolic and digestive. *Metabolic enzymes* direct nearly every chemical transaction that takes place in the cells of our bodies. They control the building of tissues and bodily fluids, detoxification, transportation of nutrients into and wastes out of cells, and much more. Each enzyme handles one single step in a series of reactions. If we are deficient in just one enzyme, the chain is broken and disease can result.

You may have discussed your liver enzymes with your doctor after a blood test. Elevation of these enzymes might indicate a disease process or a negative effect of a drug. Proper monitoring of these enzymes is important to your health. However, these enzyme tests do not reflect whether the liver is performing its many health functions optimally. They also do not measure the thousands of other metabolic enzymes that are supposed to be operating elsewhere in the body.

With precious few exceptions, there is no substitute for our body's own production of metabolic enzymes. (Only the important antioxidant enzymes glutathione peroxidase, catalase, and superoxide dismutase are available as supplements. Supplementing with colostrum greatly boosts those enzymes.) However, we can give our metabolic enzymes a boost by improving our nutrition and supplementing digestive enzymes. By better supplying the raw materials and energy required for their manufacture, these steps assist the production of metabolic enzymes. This indirectly reduces the workload for metabolic enzymes, enabling them to perform more efficiently. In addition, you will read on page 69 how supplemental enzymes can be used to control the growth of organisms in the body.

Digestive Enzymes

Digestive enzymes are vital to digestion because they direct the action. Most of us have been taught the importance of good nutrition from a young age. Yet the presence of digestive enzymes is just as important as what you eat. Consuming wonderfully nutritious food avails us nothing if we are then unable to fully digest and assimilate and/or excrete the components. Your body has different enzymes to digest different types of foods.

The body is truly amazing. It only makes the amount and type of enzymes it needs, a principle known as *adaptive secretion*. That efficiency depends on signals that are sent to indicate the type of food in the system. One of my concerns regarding acid blockers is that they interfere with that signaling and provide more work for the digestive system. It is estimated that up to 80 percent of the body's energy is used for digestion. Therefore, it stands to reason that *not* adding to the body's workload would benefit the process of digestion.

The small intestine is where the heavy lifting of enzyme digestion takes place. The intestinal lining itself releases many enzymes that digest various peptides, carbohydrates, and fats. Additionally, the pancreas gland sends the many enzymes it produces to the small intestines. These enzymes are also involved in digesting all three classes of food: proteins, fats, and carbohydrates.

Enzymes are released throughout the digestive process with the sole purpose of digesting a particular type of food. If people are intolerant (sensitive or allergic) of a certain food, it may be because they are missing or are deficient in one of the specific enzymes needed to process that food.

Protein

Protease enzymes, with the help of stomach acid, allow the body to pull peptides out of protein and digest amino acids so that they can be used to make neurotransmitters, hormones, and more enzymes. If the body doesn't have enough acid and protease when eating a meal containing meat, the protein will rot and create disgustingly foul-smelling break-down compounds with names like Putrescine and Cadaverine. Then, instead of obtaining the much-needed amino acids, we absorb these nasty toxic chemicals. If you generate particularly foul-smelling gas, you may not be properly digesting proteins.

A *peptide* is a compound made of two or more amino acids. It may take several enzymes to break down a protein into its amino acid parts because each peptide group is associated with specialized enzymes. *Pepsin* is an important enzyme found in the stomach that breaks proteins into peptides, continuing the work started by the stomach acid.

Damage to the integrity of the intestinal lining hampers our ability to create *peptidases*—enzymes to digest specific peptides—and may result in negative intestinal reactions to some proteins (such as the casein in milk or the gluten in grain). Worse yet, the resulting small particles of incompletely digested protein can leak into the bloodstream through gaps between cells of the intestinal lining and may contribute to autoimmune problems.

Fats

The health aspects of fats (lipids) will be described in greater detail in Chapter 9. For now, it is important to understand that some fats are not only good, but essential for good health. Fats must be consumed, broken down, and absorbed by the body. Stomach acid and *lipase* enzymes are both required for this process and also to release fat-soluble vitamins such as vitamins A, D, and E. When fats are consumed but not digested, they can become rancid. Rancid fats cause free radical damage to cells and speed us along the track to heart disease and cancer. Floating stools and dry skin are possible signs that fats are not being properly digested.

Carbohydrates

The digestion of carbohydrates provides the body with energy. Vegetables, fruits, grains, and beans are examples of carbohydrate foods (although they may also contain some small amounts of proteins and fats). Besides releasing energy, proper digestion of these foods also liberates the carbohydrates' vitamins, minerals, and powerful *phytonutrients*—plant compounds that protect us from inflammation and cancer. However, if not digested, the carbohydrates can be fermented by organisms in the intestines and cause bloating and noisy gas. The gas also exerts pressure back up the system. If all the valves aren't working properly, this can force digestive juices into places they don't belong, such as past the LES, and cause heartburn.

Simple sugars like table sugar need little digestion. They are therefore easily absorbed and raise the blood sugar very quickly. Digestion of starch (such as white flour) is just slightly more complex than sugar. An enzyme in saliva, *amylase*, quickly turns starch into sugar. (To observe this reaction, hold some flour in your mouth and observe the sweetness.) The more complex carbohydrates are operated on by enzymes named *disaccharidases*. One of those, *lactase*, is the enzyme that works on the carbohydrate component of milk, which is called lactose. Digestion of cellulose—the structural part of plants—requires *cellulase*, an enzyme that is produced not by our digestive systems but by our good bugs (mainly bacteria).

As you may have noticed, most enzyme names end in the suffix "ase." This information can help clarify food labels. Likewise, sugars are identified with "ose" at the end of their names and alcohols with "ol."

ENZYME DEFICIENCY AND SUPPLEMENTATION

Some people's bodies do not produce sufficient enzymes. Other people may have enough enzymes, but they may not be activated because of a lack of cofactors. This section will focus on why your body may not have sufficient enzymes, and what you can do to remedy the situation.

Causes of Enzyme Insufficiency

There are several explanations behind insufficient enzyme production or action. The first is that enzyme production decreases as we age. Some estimates claim that our enzyme production declines by approximately 10 percent each decade after our teenage years.

In addition to age, enzyme insufficiency can also be attributed to problems with the intestinal lining, where many enzymes are manufactured.

Another possible problem is inadequate dietary protein or lack of acid to digest protein. This can reduce the raw material available from which to make enzymes. Low stomach acid can also cause insufficient production of enzymes by interfering with the signaling that calls for their creation.

The enzymes that are present may simply remain inactive. The acidity/alkalinity of the area where the enzyme is to function is crucial to whether it will do its job. If stomach acid is low (either naturally or because of acid-blocking drugs), the necessary digestive enzymes may very well fail because the intestines have not been triggered to be alkaline.

Vitamin and mineral cofactors are needed for the production and operation of enzymes. If the diet is poor and/or digestion and absorption has been suboptimal for an extended period of time because of either a damaged intestinal tract or functional interference via acid blockers, there may deficits in these nutrients. As a result, the necessary enzymes may be either insufficient or inoperable.

Insufficient water is another possible cause of an enzyme remaining inactivated, so it is necessary to stay properly hydrated. Keep in mind, however, that the majority of your fluid intake should not be consumed during meals because that dilutes your stomach acid. Instead, most of your fluid intake should take place between meals.

Our beneficial gut bacteria help make hundreds of our enzymes. For example, they make the enzyme cellulase, which is required to digest plant cellulose. But, as will be discussed later, we can't take the presence of these bacteria for granted. In fact, we should do what we can to assist them in the digestive process so that they can make enzymes and perform dozens of other jobs more effectively.

Symptoms of an Enzyme Insufficiency

Each person's genetic background, diet, environment, and habits are unique. Similarly, the symptoms of having insufficient enzymes can also differ from one person to the next. Heartburn is one common sign. Another is undigested food visible in the stool, which can indicate that food is passing through the system without being fully digested.

Floating stools may be a sign of enzyme insufficiency as well, because they suggest that nutrients are passing through the digestive system unabsorbed. These nutrients then provide food for intestinal organisms that give off gas, making the stool float.

People who have not been diagnosed as allergic to milk or wheat and yet experience unpleasant reactions to them, such as gas or rashes, may not have the enzymes to properly digest them. Another person's clue to enzyme need might be depression, hormonal swings, muscle weakness, or irritable bowels.

The range of symptoms potentially generated by a deficiency of enzymes is so very broad and the risk to supplementation of enzymes so small that often natural health professionals just recommend a practical trial. Before beginning to take enzymes, you may want to make a list of all the symptoms that you experience so that you can later recognize what has improved.

Enzymes and Our Eating Habits

In addition to the enzymes produced in our bodies, we should also utilize enzymes built into food. When placed in the right environment, raw foods will literally digest themselves. We have all seen the brown spots that appear on fruit when it has been bruised. The brown shows the work of enzymes beginning to digest the fruit. This digestion encourages the plant's eventual reproduction by exposing its seeds to soil and the other elements needed for sprouting. When we chew these foods, these same enzymes are released and go right to work on the food substance.

However, most of us do not eat any significant part of our diet raw, and cooking deactivates enzymes. As a result, the burden of digestion then falls on our body's production of enzymes. Dr. Frances Pottenger studied four generations of cats and the effects of eating cooked and processed foods versus raw and natural foods. The rather dramatic results showed that the generations of felines fed a cooked and processed diet had more diseases, such as arthritis and diabetes, and shorter life spans than those that ate a more natural diet. Eating a totally raw diet is not practical and perhaps not desirable for everyone, but heartburn often clears up if a substantial part of the diet is altered to be raw. It would be rare, for example, for someone to get heartburn from eating a raw carrot.

Take smaller bites and chew more thoroughly. This will allow more food particles to be exposed to your enzymes and encourage more efficient digestion.

Relief from Enzyme Supplementation

Many people find that supplementing digestive enzymes brings fast relief from heartburn because it goes to the heart of the problem, which is that their food was not being properly digested. You have read that when food is not properly digested, it can cause a vicious cycle in which the proper nutrients and energy are not acquired, and then stomach acid and enzymes cannot be created. Enzyme supplementation can reverse this cycle by allowing food to be fully digested.

With plant-source enzymes at work dissolving consumed food in the upper part of the stomach, the body is less likely to send out a signal for more digestive fluids, which increases the bulk of liquid in the stomach. This extra liquid, combined with the extra time the mixture is in the stomach, increases the odds that the contents can get into the esophagus and cause heartburn. When we walk, bend over, lie down, or lift heavy weights, we risk allowing the stomach contents into the esophagus. In short, digestive enzymes speed the process of emptying so that the contents are less likely to travel upward.

Carbohydrates that are not fully digested may ferment. This creates alcohol and bubbles that can get into the esophagus. Common broad spectrum enzyme supplements address this by helping to digest the carbohydrate component of the meal you consumed.

Some people are allergic or sensitive to certain foods. However, foods do not cause trouble if they are *fully* digested. Therefore, enzyme supplementation can often bring relief from food "allergies," as Chapter 8 will explain.

Types of Enzyme Supplements

A general digestive enzyme will likely help your digestive process and will certainly do no harm. If you have heartburn, this is a very safe treatment to try first. It is even safer than adding HCl and much safer than blocking stomach acid. There are two basic types of supplemental enzymes: those from animal sources and those from plant sources.

I suggest to start with the enzyme supplementation Super Enzyme Caps by Twinlab. This old standby is widely available in health food stores. It is a combination of Betaine HCl, pancreatin (the most common enzyme derived from animals), and some plant enzymes. It does not contain enough acid to solve a severe shortage, but because the product contains a variety of substances, it is a reasonable starting point. Vegetarians should most likely stick with plant-source supplements. Digestive enzyme supplements should be taken at the beginning of a meal.

Enzyme Supplements from Animal Sources

Pancreatin is a collection of enzymes produced by the pancreas. It assists with the breakdown of fats, proteins, and carbohydrates. Pancreatin is the most common enzyme supplement derived from animals. When taken as a supplement, these enzymes are quite sensitive to pH changes and may not survive stomach acid unless they are *enteric-coated*—covered with an outside layer that will not dissolve until it reaches the alkaline environment of the small intestine. On the other hand, if the stomach acid is insufficient, the pancreas may not be signaled to put out enough bicarbonate, which is the substance that causes the alkalinity of the small intestine. As a result, the pH of the contents of the small intestine may not activate supplemental pancreatin under these conditions.

For purely digestive purposes, the plant-based enzymes (which are discussed in the following section) are more stable over a wider pH range than those derived from animal sources. However, I believe that animal enzymes may have the added benefit of producing a "glandular" effect. For untold centuries, people seem to have intuitively known that glands from animals can somehow assist the gland of the human who consumed it. Therefore, if you have a pancreatic problem, you may want to try the animal pancreatin first. You might even combine it with a plant source enzyme. If your pancreas is struggling, you will certainly want to support it any way you can because it is an unbelievably complex and indispensable organ.

Responsible manufacturers make certain that their supplements are free of any diseases that might be of concern to humans. The usual sources are pig or cow pancreas glands, so be aware if you have an allergy to either source.

Enzyme Supplements from Plant Sources

There are two main types of enzyme supplements derived from plants. In his book *Enzymes: What the Experts Know,* Tom Bohager says that plant enzymes are significantly stronger than animal enzymes. He states that they break down 10 to 100 times more of the same material.

The most common supplements are enzymes created by organisms, usually a fungus variety called aspergillus. Although these enzymes might be inactivated temporarily in the lower part of the stomach because of the high acid content, they are often quite effective in the upper part of the stomach and become activated again after leaving the stomach. There is no concern about sensitivity to the source material as there can be with animal or fruit enzymes.

Some fruits contain protein-digesting enzymes. For example, papain from papaya is used as a meat tenderizer and digestive aid. Chewable papaya tablets, available from health food stores in a handy pocket roll, would be a much better remedy for heartburn than an antacid. Supplements from bromelain extracted from pineapple cores are often used not so much for digestion but taken between meals to reduce inflammation and swelling somewhere in the body. I've seen the chewable variety literally digest away a bruise. However, chewing a bromelain tablet that was intended for swallowing feels very weird because it removes the layer of dead cells from your taste buds. (That is a voice of experience speaking.) They do not damage healthy tissue, but I recommend using a product designed as a chewable. There are less common enzymes that have been extracted from figs and kiwi. These fruit-based enzymes can be useful but may be less successful at improving flawed digestion, so consider the purpose for which you are taking the supplements before you pick one. You should avoid these fruit-based tablets if you are allergic to the source plant.

Selecting and Using Enzyme Supplements

Unless you are taking an enzyme supplement for a very specific purpose (such as digesting milk), broader spectrum combination blends are the better option. For example, if you believe you have a problem digesting proteins because your symptoms appear worse after eating meat, you may actually need help digesting other foods as well. Therefore, I would suggest a product that digests proteins, fats, and carbohydrates, because it will improve overall digestive function.

You should also begin your enzyme supplementation regimen slowly. Start with less than the label directions suggest. Then, add to this dosage until your symptoms are relieved. Some products may kill off organisms and digest debris so quickly that you could experience a healing discomfort known as a *die-off reaction*. Your detoxification systems might become temporarily overwhelmed. This can cause a short-term reaction such as a headache, fatigue, or a change in stool frequency or consistency. The reactions are temporary and not serious, but if you find them bothersome you can start at a lower dose and gradually increase it. Everybody is different, and you may have to experiment to find the best supplementation for you. However, it is wise to start with a well-balanced blend.

Take the supplement at the very beginning of the meal for the best results. That allows the product capsule to dissolve and mix with the food before it enters the more acidic part of the stomach. Another option is to open the capsules and mix the enzymes into the food before you eat it. Just make sure you add it to the food after the food is cooked because cooking will denature the enzyme. Take the enzymes with any substantial meals or snacks. A general rule of thumb is that the more food you eat, the more enzymes it will take to digest the meal.

Use capsules or powders rather than tablets because the tableting process generates friction and heat, which are hard on the enzymes. Enzymes are measured in terms of how much of the food material it can digest. It may take several capsules of one brand to equal the effectiveness of one capsule of another brand. This is due to both the wisdom of how the enzymes were blended and the amount of non-active fillers. I recommend purchasing an enzyme product from a company that specializes in enzymes and has a fine reputation. Enzymedica is one good brand. See the Resource section for additional options.

Prior to taking them, there is no way to determine how long you will need to use enzyme supplements. It is likely we would all be better off taking them for the rest of our lives—or, at least, until we become much better about eating nourishing raw food and chewing well.

Besides the reduction in heartburn, you may see other positive side effects. These fringe benefits can include improved overall digestion and a reduction in food sensitivities. The inset on page 77 provides more examples of these effects.

Some people with gastritis or damaged tissue in the esophagus worry about using a product that has protein-digesting enzymes for fear it will make matters worse. However, proteases don't attack the protein in healthy tissue. There could be some temporary irritation when the enzymes remove a layer of dead cells and expose fresh tissue underneath. As stated earlier, starting slowly is the key.

Fringe Benefits of Taking Enzyme Supplements

When you supplement digestive enzymes, you indirectly help metabolic enzymes. It is also possible to take enzymes that target other health issues more directly. In *Enzymes & Enzyme Therapy*, Dr. Anthony Cichoke lists sinuses, multiple sclerosis, herpes, thrombosis, back pain, and arthritis as health conditions that can benefit from enzyme therapy. Others list obesity, hardening of the arteries, high blood pressure, and psoriasis. Enzyme supplementation taken on an *empty* stomach can cause the following fringe benefits.

- Clean up cellular debris caused by an injury.

- Calm inflammation.

- Reduce the effect of airborne allergens.

- Benefit cancer therapies by digesting the protein coating on tumor cells.

- Boost the effectiveness of the immune system by helping it digest invaders.

- Break up clots.

- Shorten the duration of a cold.

CONCLUSION

A deficiency in your body's digestive enzymes can lead to heartburn. Fortunately, this is a problem that can be remedied with enzyme supplementation. This is a safe and intelligent way to solve one of the real underlying causes of heartburn as well as bring fast relief from the symptom.

CHAPTER 6

HELICOBACTER PYLORI, MYSTERY BUG

"Red meat is not bad for you.
Now blue-green meat, that's bad for you!"
—TOMMY SMOTHERS

Sometimes we can tell immediately that something isn't good for us to eat. If meat is blue-green colored, for example, it has clearly been overrun with bacteria and/or fungus. However, foods can be harmful long before they look like they are. In the United States alone, there are more than 5,000 annual deaths from food poisoning. A less obvious factor than food poisoning—but a concern that claims more lives—is bacteria that can take up residence in the stomach and become involved in chronic digestive diseases that can, in the form of ulcers and cancers, turn deadly. A bug called *Helicobacter pylori,* also called *H. pylori,* is the cause of what is likely the most common bacterial infection in the world.

SYMPTOMS AND RELATED CONDITIONS

Signs of having an *H. pylori* bacteria infection include one or more of the following: stinky breath, bloating, stomach pain, nausea, and vomiting an hour or so after a meal. Doctors do not usually test for an *H. pylori* infection unless they suspect an ulcer—and sometimes not even then. You may want to have your doctor run a test if you exhibit any of these signs, especially if you also have any of the symptoms of low stomach acid listed on page 54. Low stomach acid may be a sign of infection because the bug causes gastritis (inflammation of the stomach lining), which in turn may impair the stomach's ability to make acid and lead to heartburn. However, the relationship between *H. pylori* and acid reflux is complex and not well understood. Some studies actually show that the presence of *H. pylori* is associated with *less* erosion of the esophagus—but, almost paradoxically, eliminating the bug doesn't cause reflux.[1] A study in November 2007 summed this up: "The role of *H. pylori* infection in GERD is highly controversial."[2]

H. pylori is believed to play a role in conditions that are seemingly far removed from the stomach. These include migraine headaches, rosacea, a type of arthritis, anemia, B_{12} deficiency, glaucoma, bad breath, heart disease, atrial fibrillation, asthma, and morning sickness. Many or all of those associations can be caused by the disruption of stomach acid by *H. pylori*. Although these associations are not proven, they are strongly suspected. If you have one of these conditions as well as pain in your stomach area, you should consider getting tested for both *H. pylori* and stomach acid insufficiency.

H. pylori has a stronger foothold in countries with lower socio-economic levels. In the United States, approximately 30 percent of the population is infected. More specifically, 20 percent of people under the age of forty are infected, while 50 percent of those over fifty years old have the bacteria. For reasons that are not totally clear, the rate of *H. pylori* infection in the United States has declined by 50 percent since 1968.[3] Some attribute this reduction to an improved standard of living, better refrigeration, and access to fruits and vegetables.

The *H. pylori* bugs live in the stomach and the first part of the intestines. They have developed quite clever ways to survive. First, while normal stomach acid wipes out most organisms once they are implanted, *H. pylori* cells use our own naturally produced urea to make alkaline ammonium dioxide, which serves to protect the bacterial cells from the acid. Secondly, they make their own lives easier by reducing our ability to make gastric acid. Thirdly, *H. pylori* hides securely in the mucous lining of the stomach. The body reacts by sending white blood cells—part of the immune system—to the infected area, but the immune cells can't reach the bugs, which are protected by the stomach mucus. The white cells then accumulate and die, leaving behind nutrients to feed the bugs. The inflammation and free radicals caused by our own frustrated immune cells may actually be the eventual cause of gastritis irritation and ulcers. In a fourth survival strategy, *H. pylori* has a creepy tactic that outwits attempts of the stomach cells to eliminate the infection: the bacteria can turn off the stomach cells' normal ability to essentially self-destruct when they have become infected.[4] And lastly, our overuse of antibiotics has prompted *H. pylori* to develop into more resistant strains.

H. pylori is transmitted orally through tainted food or water. Like most pathological organisms, its effect depends largely on the condition of the host: you or me. This can be illustrated several ways. Even in areas of high incidence of infection, there are always some people who do not catch the bug. Perhaps these people have strong stomach acid barriers and immune systems that immediately take the bacterium out of commission before it can set up shop. Furthermore, of those identified as having *H. pylori* in their bodies, only one in six will get a stomach disease or related condition. Perhaps those people who do not develop the disease are better nourished and less stressed, have a good balance of friendly bacteria and better levels of stomach acid, and sustain good integrity of the GI mucous membranes. Other people get the bacteria in childhood but do not develop problems until adulthood. Could this be the result of lowered resistance from accumulated insults like medication use, smoking, alcohol excess, and bad dietary habits catching up with them? For now, these explanations, while logical, are only theories.

It may be a very long time before science unravels all the curious factors surrounding the direct and indirect effects of this bug. Clearly, however, the host environment where the *H. pylori* lives is a crucial factor—and one over which you have a great deal of control. A proper balance of beneficial bacteria to compete with the *H. pylori* for space and food, as well as attack them by producing natural anti-bacterial chemicals, can lower your risk factor. (Encouraging growth of healthy bacteria is discussed in Chapter 10.) It is also important to take in and absorb sufficient nutrients to repair the lining of the digestive tract. A healthy lining of the esophagus and stomach, combined with good strong stomach acid and armies of protective organisms, will make it much harder for *H. pylori* to implant and cause trouble.

Ulcers

Ulcers claim 9,000 American lives each year. For a very long time, doctors believed that stomach acid caused stomach ulcers. Now, thanks to the pioneering work of Australian doctors Barry J. Marshall and J. Robin Warren, it is known that 70 to 90 percent of stomach ulcers are due to the *H. pylori* bacteria. Drs. Marshall and Warren made their discovery more than twenty-five years ago and had a long uphill battle convincing medical science of the connection. Their groundbreaking research was finally acknowledged and they were awarded the Nobel Peace Prize in 2005. (The remaining instances of ulcers are typically clear-cut cases of damage from NSAID painkillers.) If a person does have an ulcer as a result of this bacterium, and reduces or blocks stomach acid to allow the stomach tissue to heal but does not also deal with the germ, the ulcer usually comes back.

Cancer

The majority of people who test positive for *H. pylori* do not develop ulcers. Many do not even have any apparent digestive health issues. (This is one reason I refer to it as the mystery bug.) Yet, when present in the body, *H. pylori* organisms cause the double whammy of increasing free radicals while also reducing antioxidants. This may explain why *H. pylori* is associated with a three to six times greater chance of contracting stomach cancer—a disease that kills over 11,000 in the United States every year.[1] (There are other risk factors for stomach cancer as well. For example, two-thirds of stomach cancer cases occur in people over age sixty-five; men are affected more often than women; and those who smoke or eat a lot of smoked and highly salted foods but not a lot of fruits and vegetables are at higher risk.) There are two types of stomach cancer. *H. pylori* is associated with the cancer in the lower part of the stomach, in an area where acid is produced. It has been reported that a person in whom the *H. pylori* infection continues for twenty to thirty years has a high risk of getting this cancer. Since 1930, there has been an 80-percent drop in gastric cancer reports and a parallel drop in *H. pylori* infections.[2] This is further evidence of the link. Despite this connection, there are confounding factors. Some parts of the world (such as Africa and India) experience high rates of *H. pylori* but low rates of stomach cancer. I propose that this advantage may be attributed to their habits of eating less sugar, adding herbs and spices to foods, and/or exposing themselves to more sunshine. After all, sugar weakens the immune system, herbs are full of cancer-protective antioxidants, and vitamin D—the sunshine vitamin—is an important cancer-fighting agent. However, I have yet to see a study on these correlations. There also appears to be an association between *H. pylori* and colon cancer (which results in 52,180 deaths per year) but it is not clear if there is actually a causal relationship.[5] There is also some evidence linking *H. pylori* with pancreatic cancer and heart disease. It is possible that the diet, habits, sanitation, toxins, or genetic makeup predispose people to having both *H. pylori* and cancer.

On the other hand, *H. pylori* does not appear to increase the risk of esophageal cancer, which kills almost 14,000 people in the United States every year. In fact, according to the latest study, the bacterium may in some odd way actually be protective![6] The most cogent explanation is that *H. pylori* hinders the stomach from making acid. As a result, the esophagus doesn't get irritated. And yet risking stomach cancer and the side effects of reduced digestive function is a high price to pay for protection from cancer of the esophagus! The more sensible route is to eliminate the negative effects of the bug but also solve the problems with the lower esophageal sphincter (LES) function so that stomach acid is not able to create a problem with those tissues.

DIAGNOSIS

According to experts, the breath test may be the best way to determine if you have a current *H. pylori* infection. For one week prior to a breath test, avoid antibiotics, Pepto-Bismol, and proton pump inhibitors (PPIs). Avoid H_2 receptor antagonist medications for twenty-four hours before the test. Another option is a blood test, which can tell if you have had an infection at some point but is less able to clarify whether the bug is still a problem.

If it is determined that you have an *H. pylori* infection, your doctor will most likely need more information to plan the best treatment regimen. He may send a scope down your throat to take a sample of tissue. The lab will then culture the bacteria found in the sample and determine which antibiotics will be effective against that particular bug. Although an extremely broad-range antibiotic may effectively destroy the bacteria, it also assures damage to the friendly organisms, as well as invites the development of antibiotic-resistant strains elsewhere.

Further details about diagnosis and currently favored treatment options are spelled out on the Helicobacter Foundation website (www.helico.com). Some of these options, as well as the typical conventional treatment, are discussed in this chapter.

TREATMENT

I cannot site convincing research that a natural supplement can, by itself, eradicate an *H. pylori* infection. However, in *Supplement Your Prescription*, Hyla Cass, MD states, "[N]atural remedies such as mastic and zinc-carnosine have cleared many cases that I've treated over the years, even with no medication at all." Along with other natural supplements, mastic is reviewed below. Because of its broad benefits, I focus on zinc-carnosine in Chapter 11. There seems little question that a combination of supplements can be very beneficial.[7] If your situation is not critical, you and your doctor may decide that you have the time to experiment with some of the following natural approaches before calling out the heavy-duty artillery: multiple antibiotics.

Oddly, there is some evidence that *H. pylori* protects against opportunistic pathogenic bacteria and yeast that can appear in its place if it is wiped out entirely.[8] Conventional wisdom suggests not to treat *H. pylori* if there are no symptoms unless there is good reason to do so, such as a family history of stomach cancer.[9] A recent US study concluded that screening and treatment for *H. pylori* was cost effective for patients over sixty years old with dyspepsia (stomach trouble), but just using the PPIs was more cost-effective when the patient was in their thirties.[10] (Notably, the study didn't address the long-term effects of having thirty-year-olds on those drugs for decades.) Getting rid of the bug may reduce gas, intolerance to milk, and bad breath—likely because stomach acid production increases after *H. pylori* is reduced.

Probiotics

In the 1800s, the germ theory generated ridicule for early bacteriologists. Today, on the other hand, nearly everyone in our germ-phobic culture accepts that bad bacteria can cause health problems. But there are also beneficial bacteria—bacteria on which life actually depends. These are called *probiotics* and they will be discussed in more detail in Chapter 10. Supplementing with these live probiotic bacteria is useful for our digestion and general health. Research shows that probiotic supplementation can improve *H. pylori* control and reduce the side effects of conventional antibiotic treatment.[11] I would advise that probiotics should be used as an adjunct to any *H. pylori* treatment plan because the antibiotics also kill off our protective bacteria. Not just any probiotic will do, however. There is one beneficial bacterial strain, TH10, that has been shown in vitro (in test tubes) to be effective against *H. pylori*.[12] As far as I know, TH10 is only contained in the probiotic system Dr. Ohhira's Probiotics 12 Plus. Don't wait until after the treatment to get on them. Take these supplements when you begin taking antibiotics, but at a different time of day. If you are able to wait on taking antibiotics, you may want to begin with a trial of natural treatments that includes probiotics. Chapter 11 will explain this further.

Sulforaphane

Sulforaphane is a sulfur-containing compound found in cruciferous vegetables such as cauliflower, cabbage, kale, and broccoli. Researchers at Johns Hopkins found that this isolate was effective against a wide variety of *H. pylori* strains, including some that are resistant to antibiotics. It was effective even if the bacteria were hidden in the cells that line the GI tract. As a bonus, sulforaphane is protective against stomach cancer through another mechanism.[13, 14] This dietary factor is likely one of the reasons that a percentage of people infected with *H. pylori* never develop symptoms. Broccoli seeds or sprouts contain the richest concentration of sulforaphane. If you don't care for the flavor, take a sulforaphane supplement such as Brocco-Max from Jarrow Formulas.

Turmeric

I speculated earlier that herbs routinely consumed in developing countries might have something to do with the reduced incidence of stomach cancer in those areas, despite greater rates of *H. pylori* infection. Studies of the familiar yellow spice turmeric lends credence to this idea because the herb and its constituent curcumin have been shown to be helpful in suppressing *H. pylori*. Fringe benefits of this spice include protection against ulcerative colitis, resistance against some cancers, and perhaps even some prevention against diabetes and Alzheimer's disease. Animal studies have shown that turmeric is beneficial for people with rheumatoid arthritis. There are anecdotal reports of benefit for back and joint pain. Given its natural anti-inflammatory properties, there may be a number of reasons to consider using turmeric.[15]

One study tested the efficiency of many natural products—turmeric, cinnamon, tarragon, nutmeg, cumin, ginger, chili, borage, black caraway, oregano, and liquorice—in ridding the body of *H. pylori*. It found turmeric to be the most effective, as well as one of only three (turmeric, borage, and parsley) that inhibited the bacteria from adhering to mucus. As the authors of the study pointed out, this mode of action is beneficial because the bacteria would not, therefore, not be able to become resistant to these products as they can to antibiotics.[16] Another study used turmeric as part of a seven-day, three-part "natural" program for *H. pylori*-induced gastritis and found that it only eradicated the bug in three of twenty-five people. However, even two months after the test, symptoms and inflammation were much improved in the others.[17] (It should be noted that the investigators also used an acid-blocking drug. When I first read this study, I wondered what the result would have been without the use of that drug. Then, in December 2007, an animal study was published that showed that the more acid, the better in stopping the spread of *H. pylori*.[18] It therefore stands to reason that the acid blockers may have hindered the effectiveness of the turmeric in this particular study.)

Although human clinical trials do not always confirm lab results, there is no harm in trying turmeric by using it in your cooking. After all, it has other potential benefits and a low risk of side effects. On rare occasions, people have an allergic reaction that shows in the form of a rash. Please note that turmeric should not be combined with Coumadin.

Mastic

Mastic is a Mediterranean food ingredient and supplement derived from tree resin. According to contributors to the prestigious *New England Journal of Medicine*, one gram per day for two weeks "can cure peptic ulcers very rapidly." In trying to determine the mechanism, the researchers conducted in vitro studies that showed that mastic killed seven strains of *H. pylori*. On the other hand, one recent study suggested that mastic was unsuccessful in killing the *H. pylori* bacteria in lab animals. However, this study may not be relatable to people. Although there have not been many studies performed, some clinicians, such as Dr. Hyla Cass, report success. Leo Galland, MD, a rock star in the field of natural medicine, recommends 500 milligrams twice a day after meals.[19]

There is little risk to trying mastic if you have *H. pylori*. The only complaint of a side effect is stomach upset. It is also inexpensive and readily available.[20] Jarrow Formulas offers a product called Mastic Gum 500. (I often recommend Jarrow products because it is a company that is conscientious about maintaining quality and available in most areas.)

Garlic

Garlic is beneficial for a great many aspects of health. However, although it may be useful as part of an *H. pylori* control program, this member of the lily family should not be considered a stand-alone treatment.

One study showed that garlic oil had anti-*H. pylori* effects and helped reduce the problem of the bug hiding in mucus in a simulated stomach environment.[21] A recent animal study (on Mongolian gerbils) showed that selenium-rich garlic had a remarkably positive effect on reducing chronic gastritis caused by *H. pylori*.[22] Given the link between chronic gastritis and stomach cancer, this is a very positive sign. (However, a later study questioned whether gerbils were an appropriate subject for this study.)

Using garlic in recipes is certainly beneficial for prevention, but it is usually necessary to supplement for significant therapeutic benefit. My preference is Kyolic Aged Garlic Extract in part because it is organic, stabilized, selenium-rich, and odor free—but mostly because there are hundreds of studies on that specific product showing that it provides a wide range of health benefits.

Ginger

Ginger is a veritable one-root pharmacy. It is extremely beneficial for nausea from any cause, such as motion sickness, morning sickness, or even chemotherapy, and is well known for its anti-inflammatory properties. It should also be appreciated for its benefit with ulcers, which, as you read earlier, are usually caused by the *H. pylori* bacteria. It is reputed to have an antibiotic effect. According to Paul Schulick, New England herbalist and author of *Ginger: Common Spice and Wonder Drug*, ginger contains eleven compounds with anti-ulcer effects. But just because a little is good, don't assume that more is better. In very large daily quantities over time, ginger can have a similar effect to the NSAIDS.

Cranberry

Cranberry, widely touted for helping prevent occurrences and escalations of urinary tract infections, is also the subject of promising research regarding *H. pylori*. Commercial cranberry juice from the supermarket is not the best choice because of its high sugar content. Sugar slows down the immune system and provides food for harmful yeast. (Yeast will be discussed in Chapter 7.) Cranberry juice is quite acidic, so if your symptoms are worsened by dietary acids you may need to avoid this remedy until you are healed.

Vitamin C

When used as an adjunct to antibiotic therapy, vitamin C has benefits for reducing *H. pylori*. In one study, a 500 milligram daily dose allowed researchers to lower the amount of antibiotics prescribed and still achieve the same effect.[23] Your first thought might be to avoid vitamin C because it is acidic, but it has actually been shown to protect the stomach lining from damage from both *H. pylori* treatment and aspirin.[24] It may additionally protect the stomach from the cancer that is linked to *H. pylori*.[25] Fringe benefits are legion and include helping your immune system and helping to prevent bleeding gums. The acidity factor can be offset by using forms of vitamin C buffered with minerals.

Curcuma Amada

Curcuma amada is an herb commonly called "mango ginger." It is a potent inhibitor of *H. pylori* with the added benefit of being an antioxidant. However, it also down-regulates acid production even more effectively than Prevacid, so it should probably only be used temporarily and for cases in which there is an ulceration and the need for lowered acid. I don't know of a commercial supplement of mango ginger, but you can find it at an Asian market or online.[26]

Alcohol

A German study of alcohol consumption showed that the odds of having an *H. pylori* infection were lowest among people who routinely consumed a moderate amount of alcohol—but infection incidence increased at higher rates of consumption. These results appeared regardless of the type of alcoholic beverage. Researchers concluded, "These results support the hypothesis that moderate alcohol consumption may favor suppression and eventual elimination of *H. pylori* infection. At higher levels of alcohol consumption, the antimicrobial effects of alcoholic beverages may be opposed by adverse systemic effects of drinking, such as adverse effects on the immune defense."[27] Alcohol also stimulates acid production, and new information has begun to show that stomach acid may protect against *H. pylori*.

Other Natural Options

There are other natural remedies described in later chapters of this book. Chapter 7 will describe berberine, a plant alkaloid that can help the body fight bacteria and other infections. DGL, zinc carnosine, and the combination product by Biotics, Bio-HPF, are supplements described in Chapter 11 that are used to heal ulcers and can also help control *H. pylori*. There is anecdotal evidence that cat's claw herb, which is detailed in Chapter 7, may possibly fight this bacteria.

Serious infections, especially conditions involving ulcerations or esophageal erosion, may need the *H. pylori* control that comes from conventional treatment, but even then, the best results will be obtained if you complement your treatment with one or more of the above natural remedies.

Conventional Drug Treatment

The standard medical treatment for *H. pylori* is a program of an acid blocker, strong antibiotics (maybe more than one), and bismuth (which is found in Pepto-Bismol). The antibiotics currently in use are amoxicillin, nitroimidazole, clarithromycin, levofloxacin, and metronidazole—but these change frequently because the bacteria quickly become resistant to their effects.[28] Bismuth does have a suppressive effect on *H. pylori* but isn't effective enough by itself and is not advised for long-term use because it can cause neurological problems. Treatments with antibiotics applied directly to the surface of the stomach lining may be faster and safer. New generation double-dose proton pump inhibitors have not been show to achieve better eradication rates than their predecessors, and they generate more side effects.[29] I believe the acid-blocking medications are unnecessary (except in cases of frank ulceration), and eagerly await further research on the subject.

CONCLUSION

As you have read, there are different methods for treating a case of *H. pylori*. Most doctors prescribe antibiotics, but these, unfortunately, also kill protective bacteria in the intestinal tract—a side effect that can have broad and lasting effects. Therefore, many people may wish to first try treating their condition with the natural remedies discussed in this chapter.

If you and your doctor agree that antibiotics are the best approach, you have little to lose and perhaps much to gain by also supplementing with one or more of the natural remedies. The various drug approaches are still being debated, but the nutritional materials have been safely used for hundreds—and sometimes—thousands of years. At the very least, please protect yourself from the unwanted side effects of the antibiotics by using the probiotics discussed in Chapter 10.

Now that you have an understanding of the problem of the *H. pylori* bacteria, Chapter 7 will detail the problems caused by and treatments of the yeast Candida, another culprit in digestive distress.

CHAPTER 7

THE YEAST CANDIDA

"Beware of the fungus among us."
—ANONYMOUS

There are many forms of fungi in the world. Mushrooms and the blue in blue cheese are both fungi. Fungus turns grain into beer and allows bread to rise. The orange fuzz on forgotten leftovers in the back of the fridge and the yucky black mildew in the shower grout: fungi. Athlete's foot, diaper rash, jock itch, and ringworm: all fungi. Fungi can cause internal health problems as well. These range from heartburn and gas to headaches and from sore joints to depression.

One type of fungus is yeast, which appears in many forms. Yeast in the genus Candida can cause infections in humans and animals. The most common species in this genus is *Candida albicans*. This chapter groups all the applicable health-damaging fungi under the general name of "Candida." (There is one type of yeast that actually has health benefits. It will be discussed in Chapter 10.)

THE HEALTH RISKS

I believe that Candida has a much wider and possibly more significant impact on consumer health than even the *H. pylori* bacteria (which was described in Chapter 6). It isn't a new threat: Dr. Orian Truss discovered a link between Candida and chronic illness back in the 1950s. However, traditional medicine is often slow to recognize the yeast connection. Paradoxically, an internet search for "Candida yeast" yields well over 1 million hits!

Like other fungi, Candida thrives in warm moist places such as the intestinal tract, the skin between the toes, and the vagina. It can exist in these areas for decades. Candida is noticed by conventional medicine when the patient makes specific complaints or the yeast becomes systemic in the blood. Unfortunately, the fungus can cause serious trouble long before that point. *Sub-clinical* is the term for a condition that is quietly generating negative health effects. A sub-clinical condition remains undetected until either someone goes looking for it or it gets so out of hand that it becomes obvious. This is often the situation with Candida.

If you are female, you may well have felt the obvious effects of Candida as an uncomfortable vaginal yeast infection, often following a round of antibiotics. You may have seen this yeast on a baby's tongue, as a condition called thrush, which appears as a white coating. Candida can also be on adult tongues and through the rest of the digestive tract.

The indirect actions of Candida include causing inflammation, reducing nutrient absorption, increasing toxic load, creating upward gas pressure that aggravates heartburn, and suppressing immune function, as well as a variety of other problems. Therefore, this fungus can cause pain throughout the body, as opposed to just where it is located, and it is extremely important to receive a correct diagnosis and treatment. If allowed to proliferate unchecked, the yeast may cause a shocking array of symptoms, as demonstrated by the list on page 97.

Ideally, stomach acid and the immune system are able to defeat the fungus. However, because of certain medications and a typical diet that is more supportive of yeast than humans, Candida can often gain enough of a foothold to quietly cause trouble. This type of infection can be a real concern—even deadly—in immune-compromised people and the elderly. One form of inflammation of the esophagus is Candida esophagitis. It is not believed to be very common, but its growth is thought to be fostered by proton pump inhibitors.[1, 2] With the widespread use of PPIs, it may be on the rise. When it affects elderly people, Candida esophagitis is associated with antibiotic use, lung disease, and malignancy.[3] One study of the elderly found that "[s]urvival was significantly less in those with Candida esophagitis with a mortality at six months of 47 percent compared to 5 percent in controls and a one-year survival of 38 percent compared to 93 percent in the control sample."[4, 5] I believe it is likely that these people were suffering with Candida somewhere in addition to in their esophagus, which may have added to immune suppression and caused other health issues.

In people with compromised immune systems, such as sufferers from AIDS or people undergoing chemotherapy, Candida can even invade the bloodstream and be life threatening. Once in the bloodstream, this yeast can cause fever, shock, and multiple organ failure. None of us can be casual about Candida because we may be unaware as to the true condition of our immune system.

The Effects Yeast Has on the Body

An overgrowth of yeast can lead to an intestinal imbalance called *dysbiosis*. When this occurs, the yeast becomes a parasite that consumes many of the host's nutrients, compromises the host's ability to digest and absorb food, reduces the host's immune function, diminishes protective bacterial colonies, causes destructive toxins to be dumped into the blood, and allows tiny components of food to be absorbed and alarm the immune system. As a result of these actions, it can cause a variety of symptoms, including those listed in the inset on the next page.

Health Risks Related to Candida

The yeast Candida can cause many health problems if it is not addressed. Unfortunately, the related effects are widespread and can be quite serious. The following list includes many, but not all, of the conditions that can occur as a result of or are greatly aggravated by an untreated Candida infection.

- ADD/ADHD
- Allergies
- Asthma
- Autoimmune conditions
- Bladder incontinence
- Bloating
- Brain fog
- Candida esophagitis
- Chronic fatigue syndrome
- Chronic lung diseases
- Chronic sinusitis
- Cirrhosis of the liver
- Crippling arthritis
- Dandruff
- Depression
- Eczema
- Esophageal cancer[6]
- Fibromyalgia
- Food sensitivities
- Gas
- Gout
- Heart infection[7]
- Heartburn
- Hives
- Hypochlorhydria
- Irritable bowels
- Jaundice
- Multiple sclerosis
- Nutrient depletion
- Obesity
- Premenstrual syndrome
- Prostatitis
- Psoriasis
- Rosacea
- Thyroid problem
- Toenail fungus
- Urinary tract infection

Doug Kaufman, author, fungus expert, and engaging TV personality, states his belief that Candida can cause diabetes in his book *Infectious Diabetes*. It is known that Candida is associated with diabetes but, as is often the case, it is difficult to distinguish the cause from the effect. Most conventional research on the connection suggests the reverse, that diabetes makes one vulnerable to Candida. That is logical because the high blood sugar levels in diabetics tend to support Candida growth, as would the diet that may have resulted in the person becoming diabetic in the first place. But, on the other hand, Candida and the toxins it produces can upset our chemistry, damage cells in the pancreas, and cause unhealthful cravings that affect blood sugar—which can cause diabetes. Fortunately, the recommended dietary changes can improve both conditions, regardless of which was the initial insult.

A growing number of researchers, including Kaufman (as illustrated in his book *The Germ that Causes Cancer*) and Italian oncologist Tullio Sumancini, think that fungus may also be a cause of many types of cancer. They have even speculated that some fungal states are misdiagnosed as cancer. Certainly there are several reasons that Candida may be at least an accessory to—if not the cause of—the manifestation of some cases of cancer. As will be further explained later in this chapter, yeasts reduce our nutritional status, impair our immune systems, and pump poisons such as acetaldehyde and mycotoxins into circulation. (Mycotoxins are discussed in more detail on page 106.) One particular mycotoxin, *aflatoxin*, which grows on grains and peanuts in storage silos, has been declared a carcinogen (cancer-causing agent) by government authorities. Michael R. Gray, MD, has called Aflatoxin B1 "possibly the most potent mutagenic agent known to humankind." (Mutagens change our genetic code, which is a factor in cancer.) Plus, this substance has the potential to not only harm us if eaten firsthand on grain, but (like antibiotics) can also be passed to us secondhand in meat and dairy from animals that have eaten tainted feed.

In the past, yeasts were thought of as tiny plants because they have cell walls similar to those of plants. However, they aren't plants because they do not have chlorophyll and do not make their own food. Rather, they are parasites. Also, their complex inner structures are very much like animal cells. So, yeasts are now viewed as a link between plant and animal.

How the Yeasts Get the Upper Hand

Almost everyone has some Candida in their digestive systems. At very low levels, it may actually perform a service by fending off various pathogenic bacteria. (It is similar in this way to the *H. pylori* bacteria.) Ordinarily, the cells quietly lead their lives as single-cell organisms. Unfortunately, all too often conditions change: the yeasts can overgrow and change into a multi-cell form. When the ratio of yeast to beneficial organisms becomes too disproportional in favor of the yeast, the trouble begins. There are three main avenues through which Candida gets out of control.

Weakened Good Bacteria

Although bacteria often get a bad rap—especially in commercials selling products positioned as "germ fighters"—there is an important distinction between the good and bad bacteria found in our bodies. The beneficial bacteria promote good health and are in fact necessary for life. When the good bacteria are killed, the yeasts and bad bacteria have an easier time taking over. Traveler's diarrhea, for example, occurs when the good bacteria have not been able to control the bad invaders and the body is desperately trying to flush out the offender.

Unfortunately, many of us unwittingly endanger our protective bugs through actions such as antibiotic use. Antibiotics are often hailed as miracle drugs and can, in fact, save lives. They may even rid you of your stomach problem if it is caused by bacteria. However, they have been viewed for quite some time as innocuous and, therefore, are often overused (even for conditions for which they have no utility). Unfortunately, they are not and were never harmless. Antibiotics are the biggest cause of flora imbalance (disturbed ratios of bacteria and other microorganisms) because most antibiotics indiscriminately kill *all* of the bacteria they encounter. To make a bad situation worse, the disease-causing bacteria can become resistant to most common antibiotics. As a result, antibiotics can be less effective when they are needed for an actual health crisis.

I always ask my clients about the last time they felt really good. Very often, they answer that it was right before they took an antibiotic for an illness or had a surgical procedure. Sadly, in many of these instances, the antibiotics were prescribed needlessly. They may have be prescribed, for example, to treat viral conditions, including the common cold, for which they have no effect.[8] Some of my patients were given antibiotics to prevent infection after surgery—sometimes without the patient's knowledge—even in cases where the procedure was minor. Whether necessary or not, the medication can kill quantities of the necessary beneficial bacteria and start a cycle of dysbiosis. The full effect of resulting problems can take weeks or months to develop; therefore, it is rare that the doctor or patient make the connection between the ultimate symptom and the anti-biotic use.

Secondhand antibiotics can be just as dangerous because of the continuousness of the exposure. Thousands of tons of antibiotics are used in the production of non-organic dairy products and meat. Some residues of these are passed to us when we eat these products. Once in the gut, antibiotics, regardless of whether they came from a pill or were consumed in food, kill friendly bacteria.

Other medicines, such as steroids, hormone replacement therapy, and birth control pills, can also damage the good bacteria that have been keeping yeasts at bay. Acid-blocking drugs and radiation diminish beneficial colonies as well. Inhaled steroids such as asthma inhalers can instigate candidiasis of the esophagus.[3]

Progress can have unintended consequences. Modern preservatives are chemicals added to foods to protect the food by killing bacteria. Chlorine is added to tap water to kill potentially pathogenic bacteria. Pesticides are used on crops to kill insects and other pests. Unfortunately, the preservatives, chlorine, and pesticides may still be in the food and water when we consume them! And they, too, kill not only bad bacteria but good bacteria as well.

A Yeast-Friendly Environment is Not Health Friendly

Yeasts will flourish if you feed them a diet high in the foods they love. They thrive on sugar, corn syrup, lactose (milk sugar), flour, cereals, breads, and sweet fruit (especially in the form of juice).

Stomach acid level and strength affects the yeasts ability to thrive. Although yeasts are relatively adaptable to environments of different pH levels, stomach acid does provide some protection on contact. Perhaps even more importantly, the friendly bacteria that keep the yeasts under control depend on the correct acidic pH established by the chain of events that start in the stomach with sufficient hydrochloric acid. Therefore, an acid deficiency—whether due to age, illness, or acid-blocking drugs—can make a person more susceptible to a yeast invasion (as well as various other infections).[9]

Failure of Immune System

Yeasts are kept in control by a variety of factors, including stomach acid and other organisms found in the digestive tract. The immune system has a part to play as well. If the system is not up to the job of keeping a yeast colony in check, the increasing numbers and changes in form of the yeast can have troublesome results.

There are several reasons immune function might be compromised. These include poor diet, stress, alcohol, smoking, toxins, and medications. Some of these factors deliver multiple insults. Sugar, for example, dampens immune function while also feeding the yeast. Stress not only greatly weakens immune function but can also drive us to eat comfort foods—which are often the same foods that encourage the spread of yeast. The length of time that the yeasts hang around is a factor, too: the immune system may grow weary of chasing a pest that is around for years.

Ultimately, once the yeast has damaged the intestinal lining and affected nutrient absorption, it also affects the body's ability to mount an effective response. This can become a vicious cycle.

Yeast and Acid Reflux

Controlling Candida is of indirect benefit to the conditions for which acid blockers are prescribed and important for overall health. However, there is also a direct link between yeast and acid reflux, as many medical professionals have noted. I believe there are several reasons for this relationship. First, as they process their food, yeasts give off gas. (This action is what makes bread rise.) When the gas is released in the lower intestines, it is expelled as flatulence. However, when the gas is severe or is generated in the upper digestive system and the protective sphincters are weakened, it can create pressure that forces digestive liquid back upstream as far as the esophagus. Heartburn can result. At the same time, when Candida has damaged the body's ability to absorb nutrients, we may not have the necessary nutrients to make stomach acid which, when sufficient, moves food out of the stomach faster. Reduced nutrient uptake also affects our ability to keep the esophagus in repair, which can cause tissue to become sensitive to whatever you swallow. Thirdly, the closing of the sphincter is triggered by a nerve impulse, and yeast is notorious for messing with our nervous system. These factors, combined with the toxins produced by the yeast, can weaken our ability to keep the yeast from taking up residence in the esophagus and causing irritation directly. Lastly, yeast can even slow the process of healing ulcerations—which usually means more prescriptions for acid blockers.[10]

Not all of the above connections have been adequately researched because, as discussed on pages 94 to 95, conventional medicine has been slow to take an interest in Candida. The relationship between yeast and acid reflux should become clearer in the future, when more studies have been performed. However, most nutrition-savvy practitioners know there is a connection and see the often-dramatic improvement in acid reflux symptoms when the yeast is treated. Understanding the fine points of the mechanism may be less important than achieving the desired result.

Consuming Nutrients

The parasitic yeasts use the nutrients of their host for their own benefit. Although we are overfed as a nation, we are undernourished in vitamins and minerals. Most people do not have micronutrients to spare. Research shows that yeasts may even use significant amounts of the CoQ10 supplements that are often taken for cardiovascular health.[11] This is especially detrimental to the many people who take CoQ10 supplements to compensate for the fact that "statin" drugs (taken to block cholesterol production) diminish the body's ability to naturally produce CoQ10.

Damaging the Digestive Tract

Villi are microscopic finger-like protrusions on the surface of the lining of the small intestine. They are crucial because they greatly increase the surface area that can absorb nutrients. However, the increased presence of yeast causes the villi to flatten, reducing the body's ability to utilize nutrients. This greatly compounds the problem that the yeasts have already appropriated many of the person's ingested nutrients for their own use.

Leaky Gut Syndrome

As the fungus changes to a more aggressive form in our intestines, it sends out threadlike extensions called *mycelia*. The mycelia penetrate the membranes that line the digestive tract and leave in their wake gaps where food particles that are not totally digested can escape into circulation. This condition of increased permeability is often referred to as *leaky gut*.

Leaky gut is a double-edged sword. It does not allow the body to absorb the nutrients it needs while also allowing the body to absorb things it should not. For example, the weakened intestinal barrier allows the body to absorb *peptides*, products of protein that are not completely digested and can cause food sensitivities. It may also result in the development or at least aggravation of various autoimmune syndromes. The inset on page 105 describes the approach of natural medicine toward this condition.

Leaky Gut Syndrome

In the field of natural medicine, leaky gut syndrome—a condition in which incompletely digested food particles are able to permeate the intestines—has been a subject of intense study and clinical innovation for many years. The focus has been on treating the yeast, rebalancing the friendly organisms, and repairing the intestinal tract. By concentrating on these areas, those in natural medicine were able to achieve positive results in cases where conventional medicine had failed. Many practitioners use the *lactulose/mannitol challenge test* to measure gut permeability and as a rough gauge of nutrient absorption. They may also use blood markers to test for food sensitivities.

The Foundation for Integrated Medicine website has a great article by Leo Galland, MD about this condition. It can be found at www.mdheal.org/leakygut.htm and includes a bibliography of the sparse but encouraging research that has been conducted on this subject. Because the concept that leaky gut can contribute to such a wide range of symptoms represents a paradigm shift for conventional medicine, it may be some time before the research is considered conclusive and even longer before the concepts are reflected in routine insurance-based medical evaluation and treatment.[12]

Creating Acetaldehyde

Acetaldehyde, an alcohol and a probable carcinogen, is a waste product generated by yeast. When released in the esophagus or stomach, acetaldehyde can add to irritation and burning on contact. When produced in the intestines, it can cause problems systemically once it is absorbed in the bloodstream. (Otherwise sober people with raging candidiasis who consume fruit juices or other food sources of Candida have been shown to have blood alcohol levels high enough to get them arrested for a DUI!) Acetaldehyde can affect several bodily systems, including the endocrine, neurological, and immune systems. It can accumulate in the brain, joints, and muscles.

Releasing Mycotoxins

Candida cells also produce and release *mycotoxins*, which are poisonous chemicals. You read on page 98 about aflatoxin, a notoriously carcinogenic mycotoxin found on agricultural products. Mycotoxins are released by the yeasts in the intestines and cause inflammation locally, but are also carried by the bloodstream to all parts of the body. There, they cause a wide variety of concerns. In the brain, for example, they might cause depression or "boggy brain" (confusion and difficulty focusing). Japanese studies (in the early 1980s) showed that the toxins interfere with hormones and enzymes. Mycotoxins can also inflame joints, interfere with the production of digestive juices, and cause a host of other symptoms. Molds produce some mycotoxins that are used as antibiotics—a mixed blessing, as you have read. Penicillin is an example.

Adversely Affecting Probiotics

The presence of probiotics—good bacteria—in your body is extremely important for good health. Unfortunately, mycotoxins and acetaldehydes, which are both released by yeasts, endanger these crucial helpful bacteria. The role of probiotics and the costly effect of endangering their numbers will be discussed in detail in Chapter 10.

Causing Constipation

In a person with Candidiasis, the combined factors of reduced probiotics and the yeast's unneighborly habit of stealing the body's nutrients often result in incomplete and ineffective digestion. This can show up as chronic constipation, which can, in turn, contribute to the further growth of Candida.

Creating Free Radicals

The yeasts—as well as pathogenic bacteria and undigested foods—create *free radicals*. Free radicals, which are also called oxidants, are damaging by-products that result when oxygen is not completely and properly processed. They can harm important parts of the body, including tissues, cells, and genetic material. The intestinal barrier, which may already be damaged by the Candida cells, can be further impaired by oxidants. It is important for your health to obtain sufficient *antioxidants*, which help control and reduce free radicals and can be found in a variety of fruits, vegetables, grains, and other foods, as well as supplements.

Decreasing Immunity

As discussed on page 104, the intestinal tract can be severely damaged by yeast overgrowth. That is of additional concern because most of the immune system resides there—and the production of immune cells can already be adversely affected by Candida, particularly by its release of mycotoxins. To understand the effects that these chemicals can have on the immune system, consider the drug cyclosporin (a toxin derived from fungus) that is used to intentionally incapacitate the immune system so that it will not reject a transplanted organ. Naturally, if we are not organ recipients, we do not want the strength and effectiveness of our immunity to be reduced by mycotoxins.

Spreading Through the Body

Once the parasitic fungus has worn down the immune system and tricked the body into tolerating its presence, yeasts can take up residence in other parts of the body such as the lungs, kidneys, bile ducts, and sinuses. Chronic sinus conditions are almost always yeast related. A toenail fungus encountered at the gym is much more likely to take hold if we have yeast elsewhere because our immune system's yeast fighting capacity is already either busy or tired of fighting it.

DIAGNOSIS

When it comes to detection of Candida, there is a large and rather puzzling gulf between conventional medicine's interest and that of doctors of nutritional, integrative, complementary, or natural medicine, often referred to as "alternative." (I put quotes around "alternative" because it is my feeling that natural/nutritional medicine is the historical, time-tested, traditional mode, whereas the pharmaceutical system is the new kid on the block—so in my opinion, *that* would rightly be the alternative.) Practitioners of alternative medicine include naturopaths, nutritionists, and chiropractors. On the one hand, conventional medicine seems almost totally oblivious to the effects of Candida except in the aforementioned cases of severely immune-compromised patients in whom the condition is obvious and/or life-threatening. In contrast, alternative practitioners routinely look for Candida because it can insidiously hide behind seemingly unrelated symptoms. When they recognize the pattern, they treat the overgrowth of the yeast— often achieving dramatic recoveries and relief from multiple symptoms simultaneously.

There are several logical explanations as to why mainstream medicine has yet to respond to Candida infections with proper focus and treatment. It is certainly not that mainstream doctors are uncaring or unintelligent. Rather, as noted earlier in this chapter, Candida is usually sub-clinical—negatively affecting health while not showing up on standard tests.

Therefore, it can be easily missed. At the same time, it is quite time-consuming for doctors to first diagnose the problem and then teach patients how to deal with yeast overgrowths—and, unfortunately, third-party payers do not support lengthy visits.

Another possibility as to why conventional doctors tend to overlook Candida may be understandable disbelief. After all, it does seem unlikely that one agent could cause the variety of chronic problems listed in the inset on page 97. According to conventional medicine, many of these are of "unknown origin" and have no known cure (which is frustrating to doctors and patients alike). Unfortunately, as you have already read, it is commonplace for the current conventional medical system to offer drugs to suppress the symptoms rather than search for and eliminate the fundamental problem. Fortunately, the skepticism usually subsides after an explanation of how yeast and probiotics function in our bodies.

It can also be difficult for doctors to obtain the necessary information. Studies published in the most prestigious medical journals have shown that pharmaceutical companies directly and indirectly control many aspects of the medical field, including setting acceptable practice guidelines and requirements for medical and continuing education. After all, a doctor can easily earn his or her required continuing medical education credits by attending a free local drug-company-sponsored seminar. Business-savvy drug companies have little incentive to teach about the yeast concept because most anti-fungal medications are past patent protection and, therefore, available to consumers for relatively low prices, whereas the popular symptom-suppressing drugs are still protected and profitable. In contrast with the frequent and local seminars hosted by the pharmaceutical companies, seminars regarding basic health issues like nutrition and Candida are much more scarce. Most doctors are not even aware of them—and those that do would have to miss time from their practice and pay their own way to attend.

Fortunately, some mainstream doctors are becoming more aware of both the Candida issue and the benefits of probiotics. We can hope that these conventional practitioners will regularly screen for yeast before long. There are sophisticated stool and antibody tests that can reveal a Candida overgrowth. But many doctors and nutritionists, including myself, often find a simple review of the signs and symptoms, such as the one found on page 217, to be sufficient. Based on the results, the person undergoes a trial of the therapy basics. This practice, which is described in detail starting below, is quite safe and offers many health benefits.

If you believe you may have an overgrowth of Candida, you should consult your healthcare professional. You may find it useful to first review the questionnaire on page 217. Your answers will allow you to form a more accurate opinion of whether you may have a problem with yeast. The quiz result will also allow you to be better prepared to explain to your doctor why you suspect yeast may be causing your symptoms. Good doctors learn from their patients.

For now, it is up to each patient to either seek out professionals with alternative training or learn about factors including low stomach acid, enzymes, and yeasts on his or her own. The best plan is to do both.

TREATMENT

If you know or even just suspect that yeast is the source of your health problems, there are many actions you can take. While pharmaceuticals—which can have potentially serious side effects—require a prescription, an anti-yeast program—which includes dietary changes and supplement regimens—can be undertaken even if you have not been diagnosed by a physician because it is healthy for you regardless of whether you are a host to Candida overgrowth. In fact, many of its aspects have wonderful fringe benefits. You may wish to check out related books, some of which are listed in the Resource section. I would also advise that you find a healthcare practitioner familiar with the problem in case you have a resistant case or any difficulty with implementation of the program.

Assist Your Detoxification Systems

When you kill yeasts, some of their toxic remains enter your circulation and create extra work for your detoxification systems, which include our skin, lungs, and kidneys. We also send toxic material out through the bowels. However, if the bowels are not open, the Candida waste material stagnates and can be reabsorbed, creating unpleasant feelings such as fatigue and headache. Dr. Sherry Rogers recommends taking a laxative (such as one to two tablespoons of Milk of Magnesia) before you start a yeast-containment program, to clear the way for the Candida residue to be quickly eliminated. After the laxative is taken, I also usually recommend liver support, which is important because the liver takes the toxins out of the circulation and repackages them for safe elimination. Support aides include the herb milk thistle or Liver Care by Himalaya (an extremely well-researched product).

Change Your Dietary Habits

Proper diet is the foundation for yeast control. Growth of the Candida fungus can be at least slowed simply by starving it of its favorite foods. You have nothing to lose by implementing at least the basics of an eating plan to control yeast because the most important changes are very healthy. Most of the foods eliminated are nutrient-poor sugars and starches that also increase the risk for heart disease, diabetes, obesity, and cancer.

In my experience, the length of time for which you need to stay on the diet depends on how long you have had the yeast problem. You may feel a lot better in as short a time as a week or two. Tough cases may take months before the symptoms really subside. Implementing all the suggestions—diet, supplements, probiotics, and the rest—will lead to faster results. When you begin to feel better and reintroduce foods into your diet, consider refraining from adding back the sugary foods. Also, watch carefully how you react to the reintroduction of grains and other common allergens because they too can have effects beyond their role as yeast food.

Foods to Avoid

If you believe you have an overgrowth of yeast, you can immediately implement the following dietary changes. First and most importantly, eliminate refined sugars, such as table sugar, brown sugar, and corn syrup, from your diet. Even real honey and real maple syrup, although marginally more healthful, should be avoided at this point. (The herbal sweetener Stevia is fine, but I truly believe that you are better off in the long run if you can break the habit of expecting so many foods to be sweet.) Sugary foods can be highly addictive so I'm not saying this will be easy at first. However, you will break this addiction within a week or two of abstinence. The inset on page 117 offers further details and help on conquering a sugar addiction. You may be surprised by how many processed foods contain high amounts of sugar, so get in the habit of reading labels.

Avoid grains such as wheat, rye, and corn. The worst long-term offenders are refined grains such as white flour and white rice. However, you should cut them all out if you suspect you have a yeast overgrowth because it seems that yeasts can live on whole grains, too (although they slow them down a bit). There is also a chance that the grains are tainted with aflatoxin (a carcinogenic described on page 98), which would hinder the rebuilding of healthful bacterial colonies. Breakfast cereals are a particularly big problem because they are also loaded with added sugar and usually eaten with milk (which, as you will see, is something else to avoid). While on this program, you may wish to use the opportunity to be observant of foods to which you might have a sensitivity—and grains are statistically found to top this list.

For at least the first couple of weeks of dietary changes, it is best to eliminate all fruit and fruit juices. This particularly applies to the sweeter juices and fruits. After the yeast cleanse, berries are a relatively good choice for routine consumption because they have a comparatively low sugar content and boast a lot of healthful antioxidants. Apples and pears are less sweet than the tropical fruits. Continue to avoid most commercial juices, which contain much more sugar than fruit and may have mold residues. If you want juice, the better choice is homemade and fresh.

Alcoholic beverages are mycotoxins and therefore hard on the good bacteria. Many also have high sugar content. Although there are some benefits to these drinks, you should wait to evaluate whether you should readmit them into your diet until after the yeast has been beaten into submission.

Milk and milk products are high in lactose, which is milk sugar. Dr. John Parks Trowbridge recommends eating a lot (two to three cups a day) of unsweetened, unflavored yogurt because it has beneficial bacteria. However, most commercial brands also contain high quantities of sugar. (Some brands that are marketed as containing less sugar have artificial sweeteners. Although they may not directly feed yeasts, they present other potential health issues and perpetuate our craving for sweetness.) Other doctors don't approve of the naturally occurring lactose in even unsweetened yogurt and recommend sticking with probiotic supplements instead of yogurt. Be more conservative at the beginning. If, later, you wish to reintroduce yogurt to your diet, be aware that dairy is another group high on the allergy list. (However, fewer people react to yogurt than to milk because the milk in yogurt has been fermented and acted on by enzymes.)

Do not eat starchy vegetables, such as potatoes, beets, and corn. After all, organisms have no trouble fermenting potatoes into vodka. That is one criterion to use as a guide: avoid foods that naturally ferment quickly.

You will want to avoid eating yeasty, moldy, and fermented foods, at least in the beginning. These include mushrooms, blue cheese, vinegars, leftovers stored too long, and peanuts. (Breads and pastries make the list, but are already being avoided because they are grains.) Some yeasty foods contain mycotoxins that will harm friendly bacteria. They may also confuse your immune system, causing what are called *cross-over reactions*, in which the immune system mistakes the fungus in the food for part of the infection. Again, it is really important to read labels because you will find trouble in some seemingly unlikely places.

Foods to Enjoy

Your first reaction to the list of foods to eliminate from your diet may be shock. It is very possible that your current diet consists *mainly* of these items. (If so, this is likely part of the problem as well as the cause of other health issues!) After all, these are the foods that are most frequently advertised— because they are made from cheap commodities and highly profitable. But don't be discouraged. The foods that you should eat are similar to the diet on which our hunter/gatherer ancestors thrived—and are extremely healthy. You can expect your energy, cholesterol, triglycerides, and other markers of health to improve as well.

Be sure to eat foods that contain protein, such as meat (ideally grass fed), poultry (ideally free range), fish (ideally wild), and eggs (ideally cage-free organic). Fish is especially beneficial because it may contain antifungal properties.

You read about avoiding starchy vegetables on page 112. All other vegetables, however, can and should be enjoyed. Green vegetables are especially healing. Although carrots are sweet, they have anti-Candida properties, according to Doug Kaufman. Tomatoes are technically a fruit, but contain lycopene, an antioxidant that has antifungal properties.[13] (Lycopene, which is also available as a supplement, is being researched as protection against several cancers, including some of the digestive tract.)

Sea vegetables are not popular in the United States but they can help the body fight Candida overgrowth. They are also a rich source of minerals needed to rebuild immunity. These minerals include iodine, which is needed to make stomach acid and certain enzymes used to deactivate yeasts. (Iodine was the go-to medical treatment for yeasts before the development of anti-fungal pharmaceuticals.) Kelp, arame, and hijiki are common varieties. They are available at health food stores and in Asian markets. Use them as seasonings, additions to soups, and side dishes because most other sources of iodine have vanished and deficiency is common.

Eat smooth nuts such as almonds and macadamias. However, be aware that the grooves in other nuts, such as pecans, may be a home to mold.

Despite possible instincts to the contrary, butter is quite alright to eat. It actually has some anti-yeast properties. You can also consume good oils such as macadamia nut oil (which is, in my opinion, the healthiest cooking oil), olive oil, and coconut oil. Macadamia oil (I suggest an unrefined Australian variety such as MacNut Oil) and coconut oil contain anti-Candida fatty acids.

Herbs such as garlic (which is discussed further on pages 119 to 120), onion, and cayenne pepper have anti-fungal properties. They can also make a diet more interesting. However, be careful with dried leaf-type herbs, as they may contain mold. (Many dried herbs are also irradiated, a process which creates unique radiolytic byproducts of unknown effect.)

Water is the best beverage you can drink. Some experts recommend drinking lots of water because it helps flush out toxins. However, be aware that unfiltered tap water contains chlorine, which may harm your probiotics.

Take Appropriate Supplements

Supplements can be an important part of your fight against Candida overgrowth. When taken for this purpose, supplements fall into three main categories: those taken to support friendly flora, those taken to improve immune function, and those taken to control the yeast directly. Supporting friendly flora (probiotics) is so important that I dedicated all of Chapter 10 to it.

To boost your immune system, I recommend taking colostrum. It not only helps rebalance the immune system, but also assists the healing of the digestive tract and promotes the health of your body's good bacteria. In Chapter 11, there is a more complete discussion of colostrum. It includes recommendations for dosage and finding a quality product.

There are many natural substances that are reputed to help control yeast, especially in its presentation as a vaginal yeast infection. Foreign research has looked at garlic, cayenne, close, propolis, and tea tree oil.[14] I'd like to see a much greater amount of scientific research supporting their use. As I've mentioned, the whole topic of sub-clinical yeast overgrowth is not yet high on the US conventional medicine scientific radar. Therefore, most of the existing research is foreign. Hopefully, this will change in the years to come.

The supplements listed here are safe for most people. (This

Cravings While on a Yeast-Cleansing Diet

It is highly likely that you will experience cravings for starches and sugars at the beginning of a diet recommended to reduce yeast overgrowth. After all, sugar is seemingly addictive in its own right. Some people actually experience physical withdrawal symptoms. However, another important reason for the craving is that yeasts love these foods and are using you to serve their needs. In effect, they are sending out their lunch order—and they can be pretty insistent. At first, you may feel an almost desperate need for sweets and starches. Fortunately, you will see a dramatic lessening of these cravings after a few days away from these carbohydrates, and most symptoms will probably dissipate when you have abstained from these foods for two weeks. Many people find that supplementing with minerals, especially chromium and vanadium, reduces cravings. These help to balance blood sugar and avoid those energy slumps. If you are used to dessert after dinner, try eating a few almonds instead. They will help take the edge off a bit at the beginning of the program. After you are weaned from sugar, you may be surprised to find that almonds are a lot sweeter than you thought. Do not let your blood sugar drop too low or you may feel compelled to grab whatever is in the vending machine to get rid of that desperate fading sensation. My clients usually have good results with "preventive eating": spacing meals to avoid a crash and carrying some protein food when away from home.

does not necessarily include pregnant women, because few supplements have been tested during pregnancy.) The inset on page 122 includes supplements that may be useful for fighting Candida but should be used with particular caution. The inset on page 126, on the other hand, describes a supplement that should *not* be used to fight Candida.

Enzymes

You may recall from Chapter 5 that enzymes are catalysts that have many functions, including helping the body digest substances. The cell walls of yeasts are made from cellulose and chitin, materials not shared by our human cells or by the cells of our friendly bacteria. This creates a great opportunity. We can go after the yeasts with enzymes that dissolve the yeasts' cell walls without bothering the cells of the digestive tract or those of the probiotics. Then, while unprotected by cell walls, the rest of the yeast cell contents can be dissolved with protein-digesting enzymes. Yeasts cannot become resistant to this type of approach. See the Resource section for suggestions on specific products.

Caprylic Acid

Caprylic acid is a medium-chain fatty acid found in coconut oil, palm oil, and butterfat. This, rather than anti-fungal medications, is the first choice of many clinics. You will get some of caprylic acid's anti-microbial benefits by using these fats in cooking. However, those oils are almost entirely saturated fats, so I recommend taking this supplement in the form of tablets or capsules. (Macadamia nut oil is still the best choice for cooking. It contains mostly healthful monounsaturated fat while also containing lauric, oleic, and palmitic fatty acid, which have properties similar to caprylic acid. For therapeutic strength, however, you may want to supplement your macademia nut oil intake with caprylic acid capsules.)

The mechanism by which caprylic acid works is unknown, but one idea is that it helps break down the cell wall of the yeast. That being the case, you may see synergistic benefits if you take both caprylic acid and enzyme products.

Some professionals recommend getting caprylic acid in the form of an enteric-coated tablet or capsule so that the pill breaks down later in the intestinal tract, where the bulk of the yeast resides. Other experts, however, believe that allowing some of the absorption to take place prior to entrance to the intestines is beneficial. This way, it can attack yeast hiding elsewhere in the body.

Although improvement in symptoms may be seen very quickly, it may take three to four months of use to achieve the desired results. Most experts recommend taking caprylic acid with food that contains fat. If you have ulcerative colitis, you should check with your health professional before trying caprylic acid.

Garlic

A popular folk remedy, garlic is recognized as beneficial for a vast variety of ailments. The "stinking rose" has many interesting constituents and we don't yet know all of its healthful benefits. Garlic can help sufferers from Candida because it is effective as an antifungal agent. One study showed that a component (DAD) killed yeast cells by creating oxidative stress in the cells.[15] Happily, garlic is an antioxidant for human cells and has fringe benefits for heart health and much more.

Raw garlic is powerful but can be irritating to the stomach. Cooked garlic is less irritating, but has a rather strong odor. With hundreds of studies to its credit, Kyolic-aged garlic is one of the most recommended forms and is odor free. I prefer the liquid form for assuring adequate dosage and good value. For women with vaginal candidiasis, liquid garlic can be added to a douche. It can also be dripped directly into the nose for help with chronic sinus issues.

Pau d'Arco

Also known as taheebo and lapacho, pau d'arco is made from the inner bark of a tropical tree and is used to make extracts and teas. It has a rich folk lore reputation for treating infections and GI problems. Modern science has also looked at its cancer-fighting properties,[16] and a tea from its bark is useful for vaginitis.[17] The trick is finding products that actually contain lapachol, the organic compound responsible for the antibiotic action, because some companies sell worthless sawdust from random rainforest trees. (Tabebuia avellanedae is the correct species.) Stick with companies that have reputations for good quality, such as Nature's Way and Source Naturals. Consult your doctor if you are on an anticoagulant medication because pau d'arco can intensify the blood-thinning effects. I have found the tea form most effective in fighting Candida overgrowth.

Berberine

Berberine is a constituent of the herbs goldenseal, barberry root, Oregon grape, and coptis, a Chinese herb. It fights Candida overgrowth and has some effect on parasites like Giardia. It also soothes inflammation of mucous membranes. Berberine has been shown to limit the oxidation of LDL cholesterol (and therefore may have a cardiovascular protective effect), support the liver, and help normalize blood sugar. To be on the safe side, allow some hours between taking it and a probiotic. It can be found as capsules, tinctures, or teas, but be aware that different products have varying amounts of the active ingredient. Some inexpensive products may not have meaningful amounts. Candibactin in the professional line Metagenics and Phytobiotic in the commercial label Enzymatic Therapy are both good choices. Follow label directions. There is also a combination product from Biotics Research that is listed in Chapter 11 and includes berberine.

Aloe Vera

Mannose is a component of aloe vera that helps keep Candida from adhering to intestinal cells.[18] It is also used for general GI distress. Among other uses, it helps heal ulcerations.

Cat's Claw

Cat's claw, also known as uña de gato, is the herb Uncaria tomentosa. There is a lot of testimonial support for its antibacterial and antifungal action, but most research has studied its reputed anti-inflammatory and immune-boosting properties. It is believed that this herb is relatively safe and has fringe benefits, so you may want to try it. Avoid taking cat's claw during pregnancy because it has not been studied in that context (which is true of most products).

Homeopathic Remedies

Despite all your best efforts with various herbs and medications, you may need to give your immune system a wake-up call if the yeasts have been present in your system for a long time. Homeopathic remedies are extremely diluted preparations, rather like immunizations, and are well suited for sending this kind of message. They are very safe. See the Resources for suggestions.

Take a Medication

Many substances are toxic to fungus. The trick is finding one

Yeast-Fighting Supplements to Be Used with Caution

The following supplements have been used to successful reduce yeast overgrowth. As you will read, they may have negative effects on other parts of your health—unlike the supplements described on pages 118 to 119, which have mainly fringe benefits. However, you may be able to avoid some of the potential negative effects of the following products by using them cautiously.

Oregano Oil

Oregano oil is an herbal extract that contains the phenolic compounds carvacrol and thymol, which have been shown to kill a wide range of fungi, protozoal parasites, and bacteria.[19] Caution is needed because it is extremely effective at eliminating bacteria—and there is no evidence that it does not kill our much-needed friendly bacteria as well. One expert told me that he inadvertently totally sterilized his system with oregano oil. For this reason, you should be careful not to overdo your oregano intake. You should also consume it at a time of day several hours removed from your probiotic supplements.

I like the oregano oil ADP from Biotics Research. It is emulsified and therefore has more surface area by which to reach yeasts. It is also sustained release, which allows it to kill yeasts located all along the system. In studies, the main side effect complaint was fatigue, but that was probably a die-off reaction.[20, 21] (A die-off reaction is a possible effect of quickly killing off many negative organisms. It usually lasts only a short time and is discussed further on page 123.) Oregano is so effective at killing organisms that the die-off reaction can be a consideration. If you want to use a liquid oregano oil, start with as little as one drop diluted in water because it can be irritating. Oregano oil should not be used in large quantities over a long period of time.

Colloidal Silver

Colloidal silver products are tiny particles of the metal silver that are suspended in liquid and effective against hundreds of organisms. No organism can survive more than moments in the presence of silver nor become resistant to it. Naturally, that creates an issue because friendly bacteria are killed as well, so take it at a different time than probiotics. According to the National Institute of Health's National Center for Complementary and Alternative Medicine, "Colloidal silver can cause serious side effects. One is Argyria, a bluish-gray discoloration of the body. Argyria is not treatable or reversible." So be very careful not to use excess amounts of colloidal silver, as well as not to use it for very long.

that doesn't also kill you or your much-needed friendly bacteria.

Depending on the condition of your liver, how clear your detox pathways are, and the amount of disease with which you started, you may or may not experience a *die-off reaction*. This refers to a flu-like feeling that can result when you quickly kill off many negative organisms. It only lasts a few days, and can occur not only when resorting to a medication but also when certain supplements or herbs are utilized. (Some people even experience a die-off reaction just from reducing their sugar/starch intake.) It is worth noting that while it is rare to find an antifungal medication that has any fringe benefits, many of natural supplements have a variety of positive side effects. Therefore, I would recommend trying the natural supplements first.

Remember that, as you read earlier, acid blockers may make a yeast problem worse. They change the environment of the whole digestive tract, which is likely to upset the delicate balance of organisms.

The following is a discussion of some of the pharmaceutical options. It often boils down to trial and error, but your doctor can do stool lab tests to determine what species of yeast you have and therefore make a more educated guess as to the right drug.

Nystatin

Nystatin is the most commonly used drug for yeast overgrowth. It is relatively safe because barely any of it is absorbed into the blood stream and so most of its effect is confined to the digestive tract. It is also inexpensive, and works in the mouth so is used for thrush. However, Nystatin tastes pretty awful, and some yeast species have become resistant to it. The relatively rare side effects include upset stomach, diarrhea, stomach pain, and skin rash.

Diflucan

Diflucan (fluconazole) is absorbed in the intestines. On the one hand, it tends to work systemically and is more effective than Nystatin; on the other hand, it is more expensive, and more likely to elicit unwanted side effects. If your doctor prescribes Diflucan, be alert to the potential development of the side effects listed in the package insert. Treatment may take anywhere from a few weeks to many months.

Nizoral

Nizoral (ketoconazole) is another antifungal drug. It is very strong and not good for a first choice. However, if all other options fail and the situation is serious, such as with an immune-compromised patient, this medication may work. It was also shown to be effective against Candida esophagitis.[23] Anyone taking this drug will be asked to take regular liver enzyme tests to detect possible liver injury. It can also lead to depression.

Sporanox

Sporanox (itraconazole) is a fairly new drug that is similar to Diflucan and may be preferred for treating certain species of yeast. It does, however, have a long list of potential side effects, and should be used with caution.

Lamisil

Lamisil (terbinafine hydrochloride) is the newest medication for Candida overgrowth. At the same time, it may be the one with which you are most familiar because it is frequently advertised on television to cure toenail fungus. It is new, so yeasts may not be resistant to it yet. On the other hand, we have not learned all its side effects. The major known concern with regard to this drug's side effects is liver failure. Although rare, liver failure is a steep price to pay for improving the look of your toenails! At the same time, toenail fungus is a clue that you might have a bigger problem with yeast and should consider the whole yeast program outlined in this chapter. To directly target toenails, I recommend original Listerine (not the blue variety) or vinegar as a soak or squirted under the offending nail. You can also try hydrogen peroxide dabbed on with a cotton ball.

Restore Balance by Increasing Probiotics

The most common cause of Candida overgrowth may be dam-

Grapefruit Seed Extract

Grapefruit seed extract is often marketed as an effective treatment for yeast overgrowth and as a method of killing microbes. According to studies and facts presented by Rob McCaleb, president of the respected Herb Research Foundation, this extract from the citrus seed is not effective for these claims.[22] Any anecdotal reports of effect at reducing Candida may be as a result of the paraben preservatives the grapefruit seed extract typically contains. Please do not confuse *grapefruit seed extract* with *grape seed extract,* which, although not used for Candida, is a responsible product with many health benefits.

age to our colonies of probiotics (protective bacteria). Without probiotics to keep yeasts in control, Candida can run wild. We want to return balance and crowd yeasts out by boosting the armies of good guys. In fact, probiotics are important not only for yeast control, but also for general digestion, prevention of acid reflux, and overall health. See Chapter 10 for more information on probiotics.

Strengthen Your Immune System

General immune support is necessary and useful to both your overall health and your resistance against fungi overgrowth. Unfortunately, yeast can stay in your body for years, even decades. This length of time can cause your immune system to become desensitized to the problem. Besides digestive issues, clues to a long-standing problem include persistent toe nail fungus, athlete's foot, sinus drainage, depression, and problems focusing. In addition to the dietary changes and other remedies described in this chapter, you may have to retrain your immune system to view the yeasts as targets. Homeopathic medicines are the only real targeted option for this chore. As explained on page 116, I recommend colostrum supplements as another way to make the immune system work smarter. According to university tests, the most potent brand is PerCoBa.

Repair the Damage

Yeasts wreak havoc on the lining of your digestive tract. Your work is not complete until you have healed the damage they have done so that you can again absorb nutrients and prevent the absorption of toxins in a normal fashion. Healing the membranes of the digestive tract is important for anyone with stomach pain, whether it is from intestinal yeast, heartburn, gastritis, ulcers, or other issues such as irritable bowel syndrome. Chapter 11 will provide more information on this process.

CONCLUSION

An overgrowth of yeast can cause a wide variety of serious health problems. It is, therefore, important to your overall well being that any such infection be dealt with effectively and promptly. Because there are several links between yeast and acid reflux, you may wish to get checked for yeast if you have heartburn—especially since treatment of the yeast overgrowth quite often results in an improvement in the symptoms of acid reflux. The more you undertake all facets of the yeast control program including diet, probiotics, and supplements, the faster your progress will be, and learning how to control these yeasts pays off with a wide range of health benefits.

CHAPTER 8

FOOD CAN BE SUCH A PAIN

*"Life expectancy would grow by leaps and bounds
if green vegetables smelled as good as bacon."*
—DOUG LARSON

We tend to blame food for heartburn because it is usually at the scene of the crime, so to speak. There are abundant theories and associated advice regarding what to eat and what to avoid. Yet current research supports new thinking. Although food is a key factor in causing acid reflux, it is not for the reasons most people think. Science is beginning to show that deciding what to eat and what not to eat is usually not as simple as avoiding acidic, fatty and/or spicy foods. This chapter will provide you with important information regarding which foods tend to be problem foods, as well as advice on determining which foods are problem foods for *you*.

SUGAR

Overconsumption of refined sugar and flour may be the single biggest problem behind acid reflux and yet, as far as I can tell, products high in these ingredients never appear on the official no-no lists. There is only the occasional mention that high blood sugar relaxes the LES. Sugar and white flour should be avoided anyway because they are *anti-nutrients*—worse than empty calories because your body utilizes nutrients to deal with them. They may also directly irritate tissues. The damaged and depleted foods to which sugar is usually added are inflammatory, feed yeasts, and inactivate white blood cells, which should be protecting us from the likes of *H. pylori* bacteria. My experience with clients shows great benefit from limiting sugar and flour and at least one study shows GERD improvement by utilizing a low carbohydrate diet.[1] A great resource for understanding the deleterious effects of sugar as well as guidelines for breaking the addiction can be found in *Lick the Sugar Habit* by Nancy Appleton, PhD. Obesity and refined carbohydrates will be addressed further in Chapter 9.

IDENTIFYING FOODS BY THEIR ACIDITY

To identify a substance's acidity, chemists use a pH scale that goes from 0 to 14. The lower the pH number, the more acidic a substance is; the higher the number, the more basic or alkaline. Battery acid, for example, is extremely acidic at 0, while Milk of Magnesia is very alkaline at 10.5. Substances with a pH of 7 are neutral. The chart on page 131 compares the pH of various foods with that of stomach acid (HCl).

As you can see on the chart, apples are more acidic than coffee, but you've probably never been told to avoid apples to help your stomach pain. You may have felt pain from tomatoes but probably not from apricots, which are the more acidic of the two. As you are probably realizing, there is much more to food reaction than acidity.

Your gut feeling (I mean that literally) is a much better indicator than the pH chart. After all, you might assume that lemon juice or vinegar would be bad choices because of their acidity (low pH)—but if your acid reflux is in fact caused by low stomach acid, they may actually offer relief instead of pain. We'll get into some more specific guides, but generally speaking, if something causes a lingering burning sensation when you eat or drink it, don't consume it until your irritation has resolved. Not all heartburn sufferers are bothered by acidic foods, but if you are, consider that the number of acidic foods and beverages you consume at one time may also be a factor. If an acidic food is just a small part of a meal that also contains less acidic foods, those more alkaline foods may act as a buffer and reduce any potential effect.

Acidic Foods

If you've ever squirted yourself in the eye with grapefruit juice or gotten vinegar in an open wound, you know that acid can irritate a tender tissue. My earliest recollection of such a reaction is from when I was a kid and had my tonsils removed. As soon as I awoke after the operation, the nurse gave me pineapple juice. Yikes! If tissue is raw and inflamed—as is the case with chronic heartburn, NERD, GERD, gastritis, and ulcers, as well as immediately after a tonsillectomy—a lot of substances, perhaps even water, will cause pain on contact.

Although a surplus of acid (whether produced by the stomach or food) is not usually the *cause* of heartburn or ulcers, it is possible that particularly acidic foods will make their presence felt as they go by the sore spot. While you are healing an ulceration or severe irritation, you may wish to abstain from consuming mass quantities of extremely acidic foods so as to avoid aggravating the tissue more than necessary.

Neutral Foods

If the pH of a food was the only factor to consider when determining which foods are advisable for people with heartburn to eat, it would logically follow that foods with a pH of around 7—and therefore either neutral or nearly neutral—would be safe to eat. However, this is not always the case.

Milk, for example, has a pH of 6.6. Because it is nearly neutral, it is less likely to create a burning sensation as it is swallowed. (Milk was often part of ulcer prescriptions before the

Table 8.1. Sample Foods and Their pH Balances

Substance	Average pH[2, 3, 4]
Lemon juice	2.3
Grape-cranberry juice	2.5
Stomach acid (HCl)	2.5 (ranges from less than 1 to 3)
Gelatin dessert	2.6
Vinegars	2.9
Fruit such as plums, apricots, strawberries, and cherries	3.0
Vitamin C (ascorbic acid)	3.0
Soft drinks	3.3
Pineapple juice	3.5
Beer	3.5
Wine	3.5
Apples	3.6
Tomatoes (as well as tomato juice, tomato soup, chili, marinara sauce, and Bloody Mary mix)	4.2
Coffee	5.1
Milk	6.6
Cooked spinach	7.0
Neutral	7.0
Vitamin C (sodium ascorbate)	7.1
Tofu (soybean curd)	7.2
Egg white	8.0

discovery of *H. pylori,* and this is likely the reason.) Yet there are several other reasons why heartburn sufferers may wish to avoid it. First of all, milk allergies and sensitivities are very common and cause inflammation. Other people find that their bodies do not properly digest the lactose in milk, which can cause gas pressure that may in turn push digestive juice into the esophagus. Then, in those people for whom excess acid is truly the cause of problems, it may be an issue that milk is known to increase the production of stomach acid. On top of that, commercial milk (from grocery stores) may contain secondhand antibiotics that can interfere with probiotics, the friendly bacteria. This, along with the fact that yeasts consume milk's constituent lactose sugar, can contribute to any potential Candida overgrowth. Commercial milk may also contain an unnaturally high level of trans fats.[2] (Visit the website www.westonaprice.org for information about the benefits of milk as nature intended it.)

Alkaline Foods

Some people are advised by their physicians to eat an "alkaline-forming diet" or an "alkaline diet." Please be aware that this has nothing to do with the figures in Table 8.1. Instead, these terms refer to the effect a food has on your chemistry *after you've digested it.* Lemons, for example, have a pH of 2.3 and are acidic—but have a systemic alkalinizing effect. Tofu is alkaline before you eat it but has an acidifying effect on the body. This can be confusing, but the critical aspect to realize is that Table 8.1 simply reflects the food's potential for burning irritated tissue *on contact.* There are books available, such as *The Acid-Alkaline Food Guide* by Susan Brown and Larry Trivieri, that list many foods along with the acidic or alkaline effect they have on the body once digested as well as their long-term health implications.

SPICY FOODS

Spicy foods are often blamed for heartburn, but studies do not show them to be a bigger problem than most other foods.[3] In fact, many herbs that add a savory flavor to foods are beneficial for the immune system, heart health, and healing.

Capsaicin, for example, is a chemical in red pepper that is known to be protective and healing to the intestinal lining.[4] However, this same chemical does improve and speed up normal digestion, and although it was not shown to increase heartburn, one study indicated that it could cause an episode to start more quickly.[5] This may explain the mistaken assumption that spicy foods cause acid reflux. Capsaicin can also cause irritation for sufferers of severe GERD. You will have to judge for yourself whether spices are appropriate for you. If you do eliminate spices from your diet, be sure to try reintroducing them periodically because your reaction to them may improve as you heal.

FATTY FOODS

For quite a while, conventional advice has suggested avoiding fatty foods. Yet newer research casts at least some doubt on this recommendation. After all, certain fats are essential for life. They are necessary for the building of cell membranes, which allow nutrients into the cells and wastes out. They make the protective sheaths around our nerves. They help compose some pretty important hormones. Many of our vitamins (A, D, E, and K) as well as crucial enzymes like CoQ10 are *fat soluble*—dissolved in fat. Perhaps most importantly, our brains are made largely of fat.

I reviewed the relevant literature, and did not find studies showing that fatty foods make heartburn or GERD worse. However, people on high-fat diets do seem to have more frequent episodes of heartburn. This is likely related to the fact that fats delay the time it takes for the stomach to empty.[5, 6]

The research implies that the overall calorie content of a meal is more relevant than its fat content. To control heartburn (and rampant obesity), therefore, we want to do a better job of limiting the calories in a meal. Many people equate calories with fats—and there is some legitimacy to that concern because there are more calories in fat than in the same amount of carbohydrate or protein. However, it is important to consider that the good fats (which are discussed on pages 135 to 137) actually boost metabolism by as much as 10 percent! Unfortunately, most conventional studies fail to distinguish between good and bad fats, let alone track whether the fats have been damaged. You should focus on healthful food, include good fats in your meals, and eat with sensible portion control as well as more slowly. Also, avoid anything that interferes with your ability to extract the fat-soluble nutrients from your meals and supplements. Orlistat is a worrisome over-the-counter medication approved for weight loss that works by blocking fat absorption—and decreases the body's ability to absorb fat-soluble nutrients.

Trans Fats

Trans fats are decidedly bad for you. They are often used to extend the shelf life of manufactured products such as cookies, crackers, granola cereals, French fries, and microwave popcorn, as well as a huge variety of other foods. Trans fats are *not* essential to life. They cause inflammation, create free radicals in the body, reduce the effectiveness of cell membranes, and antagonize the liver. It is estimated that tens of thousands of cardiovascular deaths each year could be prevented if trans fat consumption was reduced. Being inflammatory, they surely have an indirect effect on digestive health. Like other fats, they delay your stomach contents from emptying; unlike other fats, there is no benefit to eating them.

The government has finally acknowledged that trans fats are unhealthy. Companies are now required to list their inclusion on their labels. Trans fats are contained in foods that are labeled as having "partially hydrogenated" oils. I suggest avoiding these foods.

Damaged Fats and Fake Fats

Fats can be damaged if they are overheated or stored too long. This generates free radicals, which can cause tissue damage and sabotage many bodily processes. Olive oil, for example, is otherwise terrific, but is fragile and smokes or degrades at a low 325°F. On the other hand, macadamia nut oil (discussed on pages 115 to 116) is more stable and doesn't smoke until around 400°F, making it more suitable for sautéing.

Olestra is a fat substitute that contains no fat or calories. Unfortunately, it is also indigestible, and can cause loose stool and cramping. Its use also keeps some consumers from eating the needed good fats and interferes with the absorption of fat-soluble vitamins.

Monounsaturated Fats

Monounsaturated fats are healthy fats found in great abundance in olive oil, macadamia nut oil, and avocados. Besides improving metabolism, these fats are widely known to be protective against a number of diseases including heart disease, cancer, and diabetes—especially when substituted for saturated fat.

Olive oil is a key factor in the Mediterranean diet. I don't know if populations eating the Mediterranean diet have statistically less trouble with acid reflux, but I know my clients have shown fast and dramatic improvements in heartburn when they modified their American diet to be more like the Mediter-

ranean version. Part of that effect was certainly due to a
decrease in generally junky food and sugar, but I believe the
addition of monounsaturated fats had something to do with it
as well. The effect may also be a result of both the weight loss
achieved by improved metabolism and the reduction in inflammation due to improving the balance of omega-3 and omega-6
fatty acids (on which I will elaborate in the next section).

Omega-3 and Omega-6 Fatty Acids

Fish oils are extremely healthful, in large part because they
contain *omega-3 fatty acids*. Omega-3s are anti-inflammatory
and can help fight heart disease, cancer, depression, and more,
while improving mental function.

Omega-6 fatty acids, on the other hand, are also necessary for
good health—but not in the levels that most Americans consume them. These fatty acids promote inflammation, which is
required by the body in times of injury. However, the body
functions best when the pro-inflammatory and anti-inflammatory dietary intake is balanced. Ideally, our bodies would enjoy
an equal input of omega-6s and omega-3s: a 1:1 ratio such as
that eaten by our hunter-gatherer ancestors. Unfortunately, the
typical American diet is now out of control, with omega-6
overpowering omega-3 in lopsided ratios of up to 30:1. This
has likely played a part in the rise of various inflammatory diseases such as arthritis and even heart disease. Omega-6 fatty
acids are found in grains and cooking oils such as corn, soy,
and grape seed. They are also found in many processed foods.
Even our animal protein sources today have increased levels of
omega-6 fats, because farm animals and farm-raised fish are
fed grains rather than their natural diet. I recommend grass-
fed beef, wild fish, and free range or omega-3-enhanced eggs.
Most people with acid reflux do not want to encourage their
bodies to become any more inflamed, as their gastrointestinal

tract membranes are usually already on fire. Plus, inflammation dampens sphincter muscle action, a function that helps keep digestive fluids from entering the esophagus.

To restore a healthy balance of fatty acids and lower inflammation of the digestive tract, you may need to work on both sides of the equation. On the one side, it is likely that you will need to reduce your consumption of omega-6 fats. Cooking with monounsaturated fats such as unrefined olive oil (used cold or added after cooking) or tasty macadamia nut oil can improve the situation. At the same time, you should eat more fish and/or supplement your omega-3 intake with capsules or liquid fish oil. Nordic Naturals is a good brand that is widely available. Another source of omega-3s is flax oil. However, it is a less desirable option because, unlike fish oil, it contains omega-3 raw material as opposed to the therapeutic metabolites *EPA* and *DHA*, which provide the majority of the striking benefits attributed to omega-3. With flax oil, the body must have the proper enzyme and energy to convert these materials. Stress, age, deficiencies of various nutrients, and even elevated insulin can all reduce the effectiveness of that enzyme.

FOODS KNOWN TO INCREASE STOMACH ACID PRODUCTION

Some foods increase the body's production of stomach acid. However, keep in mind that *excess* stomach acid is not usually the cause of the conditions for which acid blockers are prescribed. As you have read, it is often the opposite—*low* stomach acid—that generates the symptoms. There are exceptions—such as people who suffer from Zollinger-Ellison syndrome (which was described on page 16). Regardless of which side of the equation you are on, the following list can help. You can choose to boost or lower your intake of each product depending on your situation.

Bitters

Herbal bitters stimulate stomach secretions, thereby often benefitting heartburn sufferers. Bitters were discussed in more detail on page 59.

Coffee

Doctors often discourage heartburn patients from drinking coffee—caffeinated *and* decaffeinated—because it is known to trigger the secretion of stomach acid. However, a recent study reviewed fourteen other studies on eliminating coffee from the diet of heartburn sufferers. The overall results indicated that eliminating coffee did not improve either esophagus pH or GERD.[3] On the contrary, patients who do not have extremely irritated or ulcerated tissue often report that they actually feel better drinking coffee—perhaps *because* it increases stomach acid.

As with so many foods and beverages, coffee has its positives and negatives. It is habit forming. Excess consumption may cause nervousness. In countries where coffee is boiled and not filtered (unlike in the United States), coffee may even raise cholesterol. One study showed that 200 milligrams of caffeine twice a day over a week, even among young people, increased insulin levels and seemed to adversely affect insulin sensitivity. On the flip side, coffee contains powerful antioxidants. Moderate use is associated with a reduced risk of diabetes, heart disease, some cancers, and other diseases. I recommend organic coffee because growers spray heavily and often use pesticides, like DDT, that have been banned here. (Processors claim that the pesticides are burned off when the coffee beans are roasted, but the chemicals are still released into the atmosphere and still affect the health of the agriculture workers. Rates of cancer and birth defects are high where these chemicals are used.) The Café Sonora brand is organic and receives special handling that boosts its antioxidant content.

The bottom line is that if coffee does not aggravate your condition, you should feel free to drink it in modest amounts. Other sources of caffeine should be similarly evaluated, on a case-by-case basis. (However, as I explain on page 144, I am not a fan of soft drinks in general or most so-called energy drinks.)

Lemon Juice and Vinegar

Lemon juice and vinegar are both acidic in their own right and mild stimulators of stomach acid production. If they bother you, you should avoid them. However, as noted on page 129, lemon juice and vinegar sometimes bring relief to acid-reflux sufferers—usually when their levels of stomach acid are low.

Some experts recommend apple cider vinegar for this purpose. In *Apple Cider Vinegar*, Drs. Paul and Patricia Bragg recommend sipping one-third of a teaspoon before meals and holding it in your mouth for one minute to get the juices flowing. Dr. Liz Lipski recommends diluting one tablespoon in water and drinking with meals. Other experts recommend gradually increasing from there. My favorite vinegar for this purpose is Bragg's Organic Unfiltered Apple Cider Vinegar.

Milk

You may be surprised to see milk on the list of products that can cause an increase in stomach acid production. As I mentioned earlier, doctors used to recommended milk to patients with ulcers. Remember, though, that doctors also used to think that ulcers were a result of too much stomach acid—and milk does buffer acid. However, it only does so temporarily. The overriding effect is that milk actually stimulates the production of acid.[6] Although most senior Americans need more stomach acid, I am not of the opinion that milk, especially the mass market variety, is the best response to this need. If you have an ulcer, you should give the tissues a temporary break from milk and acid.

Protein

Chewing thoroughly allows your body's feedback mechanisms to become aware of what you are eating. Your system knows that when you ingest food, especially proteins, acid is required for digestion. When you eat protein foods—which include meat, fish, poultry, eggs, and dairy—the body responds to your need for more HCl. However, excess quantities of food can easily overload your body's capacity to produce acid. Moderate consumption is the key to achieving a balance between supply and demand. A serving of meat should be closer to the size of your palm than to the size of the large portions served at some restaurants.

Wine and Beer

There is both good news and bad in regard to wine and beer. Alcoholic beverages, especially in excess, negatively affect your health by depleting nutrients, adding calories, and increasing the risk of some cancers and liver disease. On the other hand, there are important antioxidants in wine. Also, overall health statistics actually improve with *moderate* consumption of alcoholic beverages. (I sense a trend. Research also shows benefit from moderate intake of coffee and chocolate. *Moderation* may be the key—you can even eat too much broccoli.) These beverages promote our crucial stomach acid and provide some antimicrobial and sanitizing effects.[7] However, do not drink wine or beer if you find that they bother you. Pain from drinking wine may be a rather temporary problem from the acidity and alcohol irritating sensitive tissues, but it can also be a sign of an allergy to the grapes or sulfite preservatives that wines contain. Beer produces belching for some folks—which can relieve pressure for some but create problems for others. Distilled alcohol is discussed on page 145

FACTORS THAT MAY RELAX OR WEAKEN THE LES

The lower esophageal sphincter (LES) opens to both allow food to pass into the stomach and allow gas to escape upward. If the LES does not close properly, stomach acid can back up into the esophagus and cause irritation. As we have discussed, this is how acid reflux, heartburn, GERD, and NERD occur. It is therefore important to consider the foods and factors that may weaken the ability of your LES to close appropriately.

Low Stomach Acid

As I've said repeatedly, heartburn and low stomach acid often occur in the same people. One reason is that low stomach acid can cause a disruption of the feedback messaging that normally tells the LES to stay tightly closed. I think other indirect consequences of chronically low stomach acid, such as increased inflammation, are also behind inadequate sphincter function. A breakdown in the digestive cascade that begins with insufficient stomach acid results in reduced nutrient absorption, inadequate cellular repair, and toxicity. These factors surely have a negative effect on the muscular ring function.

Big Meals

Eating particularly large meals causes pressure in the stomach and makes the system think more food is coming. Therefore, the LES remains open. Most heartburn sufferers soon discover that a big meal is a big problem. As discussed earlier in the section on protein, a large meal may also overtax the ability of the digestive juices to get the mass digested—which delays the stomach from emptying. The longer acid remains in the stomach, the more likely a person is to experience heartburn.

Drugs

Various prescription medications—such as Valium, progesterone, muscle relaxants, and nitroglycerin, as well as some drugs for blood pressure, cholesterol, heart problems, and asthma—are known to weaken LES function. Please keep in mind that it makes no sense to take a drug for the side effect of another drug if you could switch the original medication to one that doesn't cause the side effect. (Of course, my preference is to solve whatever the problem is naturally without drugs.) Because drugs typically interfere with some nutrients, there are probably also many indirect ways that they can worsen heartburn.

Check with your doctor or pharmacist about any and all medications you take. I recommend the book *Consumer Drug Reference* by Consumer Reports because it clearly lays out drug side effects and safety recommendations. You can also look up your medicine in one of many online databases.

High Blood Sugar

Lots of diabetics have heartburn. There are two main reasons for this. The first is that high blood sugar relaxes the LES. The other is that the excess body weight and diet that contributed to the development of adult onset diabetes may cause a weakening of the LES. There is also the yeast connection we discussed in Chapter 7.

Food Sensitivities

There are a myriad of reactions one can have to a food. Among these are increased heart rate, a rash, or a migraine. Although I have not seen a study relating food sensitivity or even allergy to the function of the LES, I believe a connection is highly likely because sensitivities can include such a large variety of symptoms. Other effects of food sensitivities are described on page 147.

Overgrowth of Yeast

Anecdotal reports and the wealth of indirect connections (including its contribution to food sensitivities) make Candida overgrowth highly suspect in worsening the function of the lower esophageal sphincter. However, I have not found any applicable studies—and worry that such studies may be a long time in coming because there isn't an entity with an economic incentive to conduct them.

THEORIZED TRIGGERS OF ACID REFLUX

Although the following have been long thought to be acid reflux triggers because there is physiological evidence that they reduce the effectiveness of the LES, they do not appear to cause problems for everyone. Furthermore, as you will read, recent studies erode confidence in some of the routinely given advice.

Nicotine

You are likely aware that there are a great many other compelling reasons to quit smoking.[5] However, an exhaustive study that reviewed many other relevant studies did not show that smoking cessation was effective in reducing heartburn after it began. Yet it is noteworthy that one Swedish study showed a strong causal link.

Coffee

Many people believe that their acid reflux is worsened when they drink coffee. If you are one of the people with too much stomach acid or if you notice a negative effect from drinking coffee, act accordingly.

Yet a review of fourteen studies did not indicate that eliminating coffee improved function of the esophagus or reduced acid reflux symptoms.[5] That is a bit of a surprise because coffee supposedly relaxes the LES. However, as noted earlier in this chapter, coffee has beneficial components such as important antioxidants. It may also stimulate the production of stomach acid, which can cause relief for many heartburn sufferers.

Citrus Fruits

A review of current studies did not offer evidence that citrus fruits can cause acid reflux. However, this could be because many people with acid reflux have already eliminated these foods from their diets for a variety of other reasons. After all, the acidity of citrus may temporarily irritate ulcerations and damaged tissue. Citrus is also high on the list of common allergens. Another cause of avoidance is the high amine content, to which some people are intolerant. Additionally, please note that orange juice has as much sugar as a soda and so would be contraindicated for anyone with yeast issues.

Carbonated Beverages

Sodas are a triple threat. They are acidic, which can bother sufferers who have highly irritated tissue. They contain sugar, which supports fermentation and feeds yeast. The bubbles themselves (even from club soda) may put pressure on the LES and push digestive juices upward. On the other hand, if you already have a fairly constant pressure in your gut, a little carbonation—preferably from unsweetened club soda—might actually help you belch away the pressure. Observe your reactions and adjust your intake accordingly, but be aware that sodas are not good for your blood sugar, immune system, weight, or heart. Diet sodas can cause problems as well. At the very least, they perpetuate a sweet tooth.

Chocolate

Much to my own personal relief, recent studies have shown

that chocolate does not cause acid reflux. At the same time, really dark chocolate with low sugar content has health benefits that include abundant antioxidants—but recent evidence has suggested that eating chocolate every single day may have an adverse effect on bone density in the elderly.

Distilled Alcohol

One study showed that the odds of an *H. pylori* infection (which was discussed in Chapter 6) were lowest when the person consumed moderate levels of alcohol, but increased for people who consumed higher levels of alcohol, regardless of the type of alcoholic beverage.[7] The researchers' conclusion was that moderate alcohol consumption suppresses and even eliminates the HP infection. It is worth noting that researchers sometimes use alcohol in animal studies to cause the animal to develop an ulcer. Anyone who has cleaned a cut with alcohol is aware that it stings an open wound—which is effectively what occurs if you drink alcohol with erosive esophagitis or ulcers. If it bothers you, stop consuming liquor, at least until you heal. If you choose to drink, please do so responsibly and remember that distilled beverages do not have the antioxidant benefits of wine and interfere with the absorption of nutrients.

Onions

Statistically, it has not been proven that onions are related to heartburn. You, however, are not a statistic, and onions do bother some people. Some people find that their LES becomes relaxed when they eat onions. Other people have a sensitivity to the food. Still others lack the proper enzymes to digest onions, resulting in gas that puts pressure on digestive fluids to flow the wrong direction. I expect that in some cases just the fact that onions have a pungent flavor calls attention to the reflux caused by another factor. Onions do contain important phytonutrients, so whether or not to remove them from your diet will have to be a personal decision, perhaps guided by trial and error.

Mint

Research on mint has found that it reduces the effectiveness of the LES. This may come as a surprise, due to the popularity of mint tea and after-dinner mints. Unfortunately, after dinner mints and mint tea should probably be avoided if you have heartburn and they bother you. Some candies may only have artificial mint but still probably contain sugar.

Insufficient Vitamin D

Although I did not find any positive or negative research on the association between vitamin D and acid reflux, there is good reason to believe there may be a connection. After all, vitamin D is important for muscle strength—and the LES is a muscle. Vitamin D insufficiency is rampant. The other benefits of vitamin D are described in Chapter 11.

FOOD ALLERGIES AND SENSITIVITIES

We are each unique individuals with complex responses to foods and their components. According to Sherry Rogers, MD, "Every food has over a dozen mechanisms by which it can cause symptoms." One of these mechanisms is the classic allergy, which causes inflammation and reactions that not only annoy the cells and tissues, but can also cause whole systems to work incorrectly. We are born with some allergies and acquire other sensitivities along the way. Common foods to which people are allergic include milk, eggs, peanuts, tree nuts, fish, shellfish, wheat, and soy. The FDA now requires better labeling when common allergens are included in foods because some allergic individuals can have life-threatening reactions. This improved labeling helps shoppers who are aware of their sensitivities; unfortunately, the informed are in the minority and most people have no awareness that their sensitivities may be causing health problems. Also, some people are allergic to foods—such as rutabagas, chicken, or lentils—that are not considered common allergens.

Standard allergists are well trained at identifying reactions to airborne allergies, such as those to pollen. However, they are often not as attuned to food sensitivities as specialists in another branch of medicine, called Environmental Medicine or Clinical Ecology. Fortunately, there are some things you can do to at least get an idea if sensitivity may be a problem without going to a doctor, let alone a specialist. One is fast, easy, and free. First thing in the morning, before you exercise, eat, or drink, establish your base pulse rate. Then take it again after you eat. If your pulse goes up ten to twenty points, you are probably sensitive to one or more components of that meal. A book related to this topic, *The Pulse Test: Easy Allergy Detection* by Arthur F. Cocoa, MD, is out of print but you may find it at a library and there is basic information available online.

If your pulse jumps after eating, you likely have a sensitivity to that food. However, you may have a problem even if you don't have the pulse increase. Red ears after eating, changes in breathing, quickened heartbeat, mood changes, cravings, and withdrawal symptoms can also be clues. Doris J. Rapp, MD, has done wonderful work calling our attention to these subtle sensitivity clues, especially with children. *Tracking Down Hidden Food Allergy* by William Crook, MD, is a simple but extremely worthwhile book that explains how to conduct an elimination diet to identify what bothers you. Expert Anne Louise Gittleman, PhD, recommends sensitivity testing from

Meridian Valley Laboratory. Patients of Fred Pescatore, MD, and a number of my clients have had beneficial results using an allergy blood test called ALCAT. Contact information for having this test done can be found in the Resource section.

FOODS THAT ARE NOT FULLY DIGESTED

Most foods that your body *completely* digests don't cause a negative reaction because they are turned into the amino acids, simple sugars, fatty acids, vitamins, and minerals to which the body is accustomed. Conversely, foods that are not fully digested can cause problems. If the "leaky gut" condition is also present, additional systemic problems can arise.

Dairy

Lactose intolerance (resulting from a lack of lactase, the enzyme that digests milk sugar) is a very common problem, with symptoms of gas, bloating, and diarrhea. It can also mimic and be confused with heartburn, caused or aggravated by the upward pressure of the gas and bloating. Some people are allergic to the protein part of milk—casein—while others simply cannot digest it.

Wheat

The inability to process gluten, the rubbery protein component of grains, is an extremely common problem. Gluten intolerance, also referred to as gluten enteropathy and celiac sprue, is an autoimmune problem with a hereditary connection. It can cause skin rashes, mood and memory issues, and digestive problems such as diarrhea. According to the *Total Wellness* newsletter by Sherry Rogers, MD, gluten problems can also cause depression, arthritis, severe malnutrition, and nerve problems. It can even mimic amyotrophic lateral sclerosis (ALS or Lou Gehrig's disease).[8] Only one-third of those with gluten enteropathy are aware of gut symptoms. Suspect a gluten problem if you have osteoporosis, nerve pain, neuropathy, or intermittent paralysis.

In *Enzymes: Go with Your Gut*, Karen DeFelice instructs readers on how to create a gluten- and casein-free diet. As she points out, it is difficult to totally eliminate gluten from the diet because it is hidden in so many foods, but there are enzymes that help the digestive process and can be taken as supplements.

THE ROLE OF ENZYMES

Even if you don't have a deficiency of a particular enzyme, such as a lactase deficiency causing lactose intolerance, you may have a reduction in general digestive enzymes, which can cause food to be digested slowly. If a meal sits in the stomach too long, extra digestive juice is produced and the odds increase that some will spill into the esophagus. Also, undigested foods lingering in the digestive tract can be eaten by bad critters and generate toxins can that cause inflammation. Chronically low stomach acid (from routine causes or because of various medications including acid blockers) may create more work for your enzymes.

As noted in Chapter 5, over-processed foods, cooked foods, and large meals may place a strain on your pool of digestive enzymes. Raw foods come with their own enzymes and will literally digest themselves, especially when chewed thoroughly.

COMBINING FOODS

Eating certain combinations of foods at the same meal can be a concern for those who experience acid reflux. Sufferers need to be particularly cautious about combining foods that take different amounts of time to digest.

An example would be eating melons with meat. Melons are

a raw food. They contain sugars and lots of live enzymes, and are quick to digest themselves. Meat and its fats, however, may sit for a relatively long time before being digested by the stomach acid and other digestive fluids. This is especially likely if the meat wasn't chewed thoroughly enough and/or stomach acid is low. The faster-digesting foods like the melon then ferment into alcohol and may slosh upward into the esophagus while waiting for the meat to catch up and the stomach to empty. Orange juice with bacon and eggs is a typical combination to which some people react badly. Instead of blaming the reaction on the acidity of the juice or the fattiness of the meal, consider that the gas, pressure, and pain might well be due to the mismatched combination.

THE AMERICAN DIET

A huge percentage of Americans eat a diet that is both fattening and nutritionally inadequate. It lacks nutrients in part because it is so full of nutritionally bankrupt items such as sugar, starch, damaged fats, and fake ingredients. Many people do not eat enough protein to repair tissue, keep the stomach in the habit of producing stomach acid, provide the amino acids required to make enzymes, and maintain muscle tissue like the LES. The standard American diet (SAD) leads to the dual problems of being simultaneously overweight and undernourished.

In roughly 400 BC, Hippocrates—recognized as the "father of medicine"—said, "Our food should be our medicine." I agree with him. We are going to eat anyway. We may as well aim for a healthful diet that will keep our bodies in the best possible condition.

GOOD FOODS

Despite how it may seem, it isn't all bad news about foods.

There is some evidence that eating plant foods helps the LES close and helps prevent Barrett's esophagus (a condition described on page 188). Cabbage juice is healing to GI membranes. Sulforaphane, which is found in cruciferous vegetables like broccoli and was discussed on pages 10 to 11, not only keeps *H. pylori* bacteria under control, but also provides resistance against cancer. For reasons that are not clear, bananas may bring you instant relief from heartburn. Betaine—found in beets, liver, eggs, fish, beans, and whole grains—was shown in a study in Greece to reduce inflammation, which can be beneficial to heartburn sufferers.

It is also important to eat a *variety* of these healthy foods because all foods have both positive and negative aspects. Even the healthiest of foods should not be eaten in excess. Too much broccoli, for example, can cause thyroid problems! You may have to take a close look at the foods you eat to determine if you are actually eating variety. For example, hamburgers, spaghetti with meal sauce, and meal pizza are all combinations of beef, tomatoes, and wheat. Even if you don't think you have a gluten issue, you can broaden your horizons by eating less grain and replacing wheat and corn with millet, quinoa, amaranth, buckwheat, teff, or brown rice. (Corn doesn't have gluten but is high on the allergy list and can be contaminated with aflatoxins. Also, we are already overexposed to it, as it is an ingredient in most processed foods.)

CONCLUSION

As you have seen, there are many factors that can cause heartburn. But don't feel overwhelmed because I'll help you find your way. There is a simple guide that starts on page 207 and can help you identify the likely suspects contributing to your heartburn. Because the typical doctor does not have the time or training to thoroughly analyze your situation and find the root cause of your distress, it will be important for you to think like a detective as you figure out the problem. This type of thorough preparation will even help you get the most out of a visit to an alternative practitioner.

CHAPTER 9

NEW HABITS, NEW HEALTH

*"Sickness is the vengeance of nature
for the violation of her laws."*
—CHARLES SIMMONS

As citizens of a technologically advanced nation, we have come to expect that solutions to health problems will come from high-tech research, new chemicals, and exciting gizmos. These products make news because they pique the interest of the public and the relevant research easily receives big funding because there is potential profit in these innovations. Yet the fact is that the most dramatic improvements in our health come from remembering and obeying the simple and logical laws of nature. While cutting-edge drugs and surgical techniques are at times life saving, there is no question that the majority of the most powerful long-term health benefits are results of consumer choices such as quitting smoking, getting exercise, sleeping regular hours, eating well, maintaining a positive outlook, and avoiding toxic substances.

In days gone by, the now dwindling ranks of general practice family physicians monitored these basics and taught patients ways to improve their general health. (The root of the word "doctor" is "docere"—to teach.) But given today's realities of insurance and Medicare reimbursement, doctors do not have the luxury of that kind of time. When was the last time a GP made an unsolicited inquiry about your bowel habits? Today's doctor typically has only two choices for a patient with acid reflux: he can dispense a prescription for an acid blocker and/or he can offer a referral to a specialist, usually a gastroenterologist. Every one of my clients who went to a gastroenterologist was given a high-tech solution—an acid-blocking drug, a prescription for an anti-inflammatory medication, and/or surgery. However, there are other types of specialists who use non-toxic therapies that are supportive of the natural laws. These doctors usually attempt to solve the root causes of your problems. As you have read, it is extremely beneficial for you and your doctor to discover the underlying issues, rather than simply suppressing or masking the symptoms.

In this chapter, you will first read about an example of one such root cause that I have found to be a frequent yet seldom-addressed cause of acid reflux. You will then read about natural treatment methods and lifestyle changes that may reduce acid reflux caused or at least intensified by a variety of factors.

HIATUS HERNIA

There are certain basic causes of acid reflux that, if discovered, can be treated with non-invasive treatment methods. One example of such a cause that is often overlooked by conventional doctors is a *hiatus hernia*. A very common condition, a hiatus hernia—also called a *hiatal hernia*—is a structural malfunction in which the stomach protrudes through the dia-phragm. Treating this type of hernia addresses the underlying problem and can lead to a long-lasting fix. You might suspect a hiatus hernia if you feel like pills get stuck on the way down, regurgitate stomach acid after you eat, or have pain right in the middle of your chest. Another clue is the inability to take a deep abdominal breath without lifting your shoulders.

There is a hole in the muscular diaphragm that helps us breathe. The esophagus sphincter is supposed to be at the same level as this hole. This allows the diaphragm to put pressure on the esophagus, keeping it closed when food travels through. However, when a portion of the stomach gets pushed above the natural juncture at the diaphragm, the pressure may act in the opposite way and not allow the LES to close properly. Food and digestive juice can then get into and become trapped in the esophagus rather than proceeding to the stomach. The esophageal tissues are not protected by mucus, so exposure to stomach acid and food irritates and eventually erodes them. Although an acid blocker may temporarily reduce the resulting pain, it will not fix the structural problem, so a reoccurrence is inevitable.

A hiatus hernia can also be an indirect aggravator of digestive distress. The abnormal arrangement of body parts can put pressure on the vagus nerve—the nerve that controls the making of acid—which in turn may tell the stomach to produce too much or too little hydrochloric acid. Both extremes are unhealthy.

This type of hernia can be caused by obesity, smoking, and/or stress. Other potential causes are frequent straining on the toilet, a chronic cough, and prolonged vomiting. The list also includes constipation, pregnancy, constrictive clothing, weight lifting, blows to the midsection, and whiplash. While these physical situations are potential triggers, a person's general condition usually has a great bearing on the body's ability to repair and put things back in order. I believe poor diet, inadequate digestion, and yeast overgrowth may be indirect causes because when those conditions exist, nothing works quite right—and they are also often behind some of the predisposing conditions on the proven list of GERD aggravators, such as obesity. I further suspect that food sensitivities, nutrient deficiencies, consumption of excess roughage, and/or yeast overgrowth may have some negative effect on the maintenance of proper stomach/diaphragm/esophagus positioning—which can lead to a hernia. Once the problem has been corrected, it is important to consider how it may have originated in order to keep it from recurring.

It speaks to systemic factors that hiatus hernia sufferers often have problems with the operation of other sphincters, such as the pyloric sphincter. When functioning correctly, the pyloric sphincter keeps material that has entered the small intestine from re-entering the stomach—and possibly even into the esophagus if the LES is also not working properly. Another important juncture is the ileocecal valve, which separates the small intestine from the large intestine. This sphincter keeps the large intestine "sewage" from traveling back upstream into the small intestine, where only nutrients should be absorbed. If this valve doesn't close properly, toxic waste can be absorbed, leading to headaches and other complaints.

Conventional treatment of a hiatus hernia is surgery. Like any surgical procedure, there are inherent risks, as well as the possibility of uncomfortable side effects and having to have it redone after some years. I recommend finding a professional—such as a doctor of osteopathy (DO), chiropractor, Myo- practor, or experienced massage therapist—with the expertise to provide you with non-surgical options. (In contrast to a chiropractor, who will move bones more directly, a Myopractor works on the soft tissues—such as muscles, tendons, and fascia—that hold the bones in place. Some may call themselves specialists in deep-tissue body work rather than Myopractors.) The treatment may take more than one session and you will need to stop doing whatever caused the hernia to occur. But even the first adjustment is likely to bring relief and allow the tissues to start healing. These professionals can also help relieve problems with the other sphincters I mentioned. They can even teach you some techniques to use at home to help maintain the proper structure. Instructions for doing these techniques yourself can be found in books or online, but although you are unlikely to hurt yourself trying them at home, I think the best results are obtained by having a professional at least first fix the problem and then demonstrate maintenance practices before you begin doing the work yourself. Exercises that strengthen the core muscles will also support the proper positioning of internal parts.

Another reason to seek professional help is that there might be other factors at work. For example, consider that all the nerves supplying instructions to organs go down the spinal cord, which feeds through the vertebrae. Therefore, a misalignment of a vertebrae can create pressure and decrease the nerve supply to the stomach. Maladjustment (subluxation) of thoracic vertebrae 6 (T6) can cause indigestion and heartburn. Issues with T7 may aggravate gastritis or ulcers. A professional will likely be able to help with these problems.

Therefore, I do not consider a body tune-up or a periodic stress-relieving massage a luxury. I try to get a structural onceover every month or so because it is amazing how a little misalignment in our foundation can have ripple effects. Maybe you sit on your wallet, your desk chair is not at the right height, you pick up your grandchild in not quite the right way, or you sit in an airline seat at an odd angle to avoid the neighboring passenger. There are many everyday activities that put stress on our spines. I had a back problem that lingered until a chiropractor discovered that I had been wearing a pair of tennis shoes in which a tiny arch support insert had worked itself loose and wiggled to the wrong side. If our structure is out of alignment, it puts stress on the whole body and interferes with the nerve and blood supply to organs. Some of these professionals are trained in an amazing and useful technique called kinesiology, which is testing of the muscles. They use it to tap into the body's wisdom to confirm the judgments they made from their observations.

Acupuncture can be useful, too, because it has been shown to help digestive function,[1] but if the stomach is physically in the wrong place, you should start with one of practitioners above. Seeing a psychologist or therapist may also be beneficial because some emotions, such as anger, can be hard on the digestive tract. Bach flower remedies, which are flower materials diluted in water or brandy, can help further alleviate the impact of negative emotions.

LIFESTYLE FACTORS

If you are savvy enough to have chosen a family doctor who sees the wisdom in discovering the cause of your acid reflux rather than just covering up the symptoms, he or she may have discussed one or more of the following suggestions with you. All have the potential to help with little to no side effects, but some are fairly easy to implement while others may take more time and effort. I'll list the easier stuff first, but consider implementing as many of these suggestions as apply to your case.

Eat Smaller, More Frequent Meals

I suggest eating smaller and more frequent meals than you may be eating now. This advice is a bit controversial, as some authorities (mainly those who believe the problem of acid reflux is related excess acid) say that more meals equates to more acid.[2] In my experience, however, patients often find that they feel better when they make this change. After all, large meals physically stretch the stomach, confuse the LES, generate more digestive juices, and push stomach acid nearer to the esophagus. Large meals also tax your digestive juices, including enzymes, which can slow your stomach from emptying. On the other hand, eating smaller amounts—especially if you also eat slowly and chew thoroughly—allows your stomach to empty more quickly. Eating frequently helps stabilize blood sugar levels and control body weight because you are less likely to binge on junk, which can be easy to justify when blood sugar is low.

It may take focus and practice to eat smaller meals. My father used to praise me for eating a lot and made it a personal challenge to get buffet restaurants to regret "all you can eat" signs. My mother, like most, believed that we should end meals with a clean plate, no matter what was served. Being calm and focused while eating, and chewing and eating slowly, will make it easier for you to eat smaller meals. These ideas are discussed in the next two sections.

Be Calm and Focused When You Eat

Digestion is tied to your brain. The mere act of looking at, smelling, or thinking about food generates the flow of digestive juices. Conversely, stress sends blood away from the stomach and digestive organs, reduces enzymes in the saliva, and literally shuts down digestion. If you are continually under stress, you may become depleted of a number of nutrients, including magnesium. A shortage of this mineral can cause muscle twitching and cramps—which can include spasms of digestive sphincters that can keep food from moving through and results in a feeling that suggests food is caught in the chest. Also, when we are under emotional stress, we are not typically drawn to healthy foods (like salads) that digest easily. Comfort foods, such as half a pot roast or a cake, might be more to our liking in stressful times.

In his book *The Slow Down Diet*, Marc David illuminates the physiological effects of stress and the benefits of slow deep breathing before meals. He also points out that there is scientific evidence that saying grace before a meal improves digestive function. During prayer and meditation, we are calming ourselves and probably breathing more deeply. Experts in mind/body medicine say that stomach problems are often related to fear and anger, so there may be an added benefit from feeling safer and more forgiving after strengthening one's spiritual bond from saying grace.

Take Your Time While Eating

There is no cost to eating and chewing more slowly, and the benefits are huge. Many of us learned to eat fast as children so we could go back outside to play. That habit was often only reinforced as we grew up with busy school schedules and careers. Unfortunately, many people never consider the consequences of speed eating.

There are lots of reasons to chew thoroughly. It makes choking less likely. The digestion of some foods, particularly starches, actually begins with enzymes in the mouth. Chewing more slowly allows this phase of digestion to be accomplished more completely and stimulates saliva, which contains enzymes. Producing more saliva is also beneficial because saliva, which is alkaline, helps protect the esophagus from acid damage. Thorough chewing—or chewing until the solids are nearly liquid—pulverizes the food so that digestive fluids in the stomach can reach more surface area of the food particles and process the meal faster. In addition, our attention to food and food components absorbed in the mouth sends signals to the rest of the digestive tract to prepare to digest what is coming. Thorough chewing also helps reduce the amount of air you swallow, which reduces bloating.

Savoring your food will allow you to feel full and emotionally satisfied. By contrast, eating quickly and without mindfulness may cause you to feel the urge to eat again before your body needs more food. Be conscious of the fact that eating at events, while watching television, or when under stress usually causes us to lose our calm and focus. We may also eat faster and eat more. Be mindful of these habits, improve them, and reap the benefits.

Drink More Water, But Not with Meals

My mother used to caution against washing food down with milk or water. I don't think she knew why, but it turns out that she was right. This applies not only to milk and water, but to all other beverages as well, such as iced tea, juice, and soft drinks.

Think about a glass of iced tea, drank immediately after eating a meal of barbecue. The tea greatly dilutes stomach acid, inhibiting its ability to break down protein; pepsin, further inhibiting the breakdown of protein; and lipase, restricting the body's ability to begin the digestion of fats. It also adds to the quantity of material in the stomach, increasing the chance that some of it will find its way back into the esophagus.

At the same time, some professionals have theorized that heartburn might be an early clue of dehydration. Water, after all, is required for the production of saliva, stomach acid, and sodium bicarbonate (which neutralizes stomach acid when it is no longer needed).

The standard advice is to drink eight glasses of water a day. I believe this should be adjusted to consider the size of the person and the circumstances. I agree with Dr. Pescatore, who advises drinking as many ounces a day as half your weight in pounds. A 150-pound person, for example, should drink 75 ounces of water. But even that recommendation should be modified to suit the individual's habits and environment. A person who eats mostly wet food (such as soups and raw foods) needs less water. A person who is physically active in a dry climate or who takes diuretic medication might require more. Some conventional medical authorities suggest ignoring these guidelines and drinking according to your thirst. My concern with that advice is that chronically low water intake can lead to a blunting of our thirst mechanism. It also seems that older folks lose sensitivity to thirst. Additionally, we sometimes confuse thirst with hunger, and end up eating instead of having a drink of water. You will just have to experiment to see what level of intake works for you. Regardless, though, you should drink the bulk of your fluids between meals.

Stay Upright After a Large Meal

You should not lay down for two to three hours after eating a large meal. This allows you to keep the powerful force of gravity working for you. Remaining upright will encourage your stomach contents to proceed further down the digestive tract instead of running uphill and burning your esophagus. Two hours may be enough time to digest a bowl of soup and a salad. If you have eaten a particularly large meal, it may take as long as three to four hours, especially if your stomach acid is low. You will have to determine what time lag works for you.

Many heartburn patients rely only on this suggestion and get relief. Although this is an important and positive step, this method may merely avoid the symptom, rather than solve the real problem. There may still be something amiss in the digestive system. If you have to stay upright for hours after eating a normal-sized meal to prevent acid reflux, you should work with a doctor to find the bigger problem.

Once normal function is restored, you may find that you can lie down sooner after eating. However, keep in mind that eating close to bedtime will cause the body's energy to be directed to digesting the meal rather than repairing body. As Byron Richards, CCN points out in *The Leptin Diet*, waiting three hours after eating before going to bed also improves the body's ability to burn unwanted fat.

Elevate the Head of Your Bed

Even a small opening in an incompletely closed sphincter can allow HCl to leak into the esophagus if gravity is working against you. Elevating the head of your bed can help. The elevation can be as little as six inches. Bricks or blocks under the legs at the head of the bed can accomplish the incline. Don't try to use extra pillows. They can shift and may send you to a chiropractor for structural adjustments.

This elevation is a good temporary way to stop damaging your esophagus tissues. Like staying upright after a large meal, this is not a cure to the underlying problem. You will still need to address the real issue, whether it is a hiatus hernia, low stomach acid, *H. pylori* infection, yeast overgrowth, and/or bad habits.

Wait After a Meal Before Exercising

You should allow two hours to pass between eating and exercising. Although exercise is a very important part of good health, you should not do it right after eating. Complete digestion and assimilation of nutrients takes a lot of energy and requires blood flow. Physical activity pulls energy and blood away from the digestive tract and into muscles. Exercise may also physically slosh stomach contents into the esophagus. Bending over and lifting heavy objects, like weights, can also be a problem because you are putting additional physical pressure on the stomach and gravity will work to send stomach contents the wrong direction.

Avoid Tight-Fitting Clothing Around Your Middle

There is a good reason so many folks loosen their belts after Thanksgiving dinner. We know we will be more comfortable if we provide our stuffed bellies with more room. This also keeps the churning mass from backing up into the esophagus. Avoid tight waist bands, belts, and girdles. However, if you practice my advice from earlier in this section regarding smaller and slower meals, you may not become particularly bloated and may not need to worry about your belt. If you also add the advice about weight loss later in this chapter, you may actually be shopping for a smaller belt.

Get Some Sunshine

The sun's rays on our skin cause our bodies to make vitamin D. Low levels of this vitamin are associated with muscle weakness—and the esophagus, sphincters, and stomach are all muscular. Get twenty minutes of sunshine a day or take a vitamin D_3 (cholecalciferol) supplement. A dose of 2,000 IU per day is becoming common. Only a few individuals have a hypersensitivity to this vitamin.

Don't Give Bad Genes More Power

I believe that we, as a society, tend to place too much blame on our heredity and not acknowledge that we have a lot of control over whether our genes express their potential. Some conditions for which acid blockers are prescribed do run in some families. However, even for conditions that have been linked through generations of the same family, it is very hard to determine if they are actually more attributable to genes or to bad habits being handed down from one generation to the next. You obviously can't choose your genes—but you *can* control, to a large extent, how they behave, by making positive nutrition and lifestyle choices. The study of how nutrition is involved in this process is called *nutrigenomics* and explains that a healthful diet of real food with adequate high quality protein, good fats, fresh vegetables, and fruits along with prudent supplementation decreases the function of the bad genes and upregulates (increases) the beneficial ones.

Encourage Stomach Emptying

According to statistics, the stomach empties more slowly as we age, allowing more opportunity for acid to come up the esophagus. We cannot control the aging process, but we can slow the decline of function in stomach emptying by adopting a healthful lifestyle and refraining from the use of acid-blocking drugs.[3] The reduction in acid caused by these medications slows digestion, and can also result in insufficient enzymes. Other changes to improve your digestive function are described throughout this chapter.

Lower Your Stress Level

Stress depletes nutrients and interferes with many fundamental systems, right down to the cellular level, and can be at least partially responsible for a great number of health problems. Stress affects food choice, speed of eating, and the production of digestive juices. There is also evidence that prolonged emotional stress can increase the fragility of the esophageal membranes.[4] There are many different causes and remedies for stress, and learning to control it is a very important step toward recovery.

Take Anti-Inflammatories Sparingly

Non-steroidal anti-inflammatory drugs (NSAIDs) include aspirin, Advil, Motrin, Celebrex, and a host of others. These medications are taken to reduce inflammation, pain, and fever. However, they break down the tissues of the stomach and esophagus both directly on contact and indirectly, and can cause chronic bleeding and deadly ulcers. Unfortunately, coated or timed-release varieties are only a tiny bit better because NSAIDs also work systemically—throughout the body—and interfere with the maintenance of membranes. As noted in

Chapter 3, Vioxx was an NSAID with less gastrointestinal risk. It was recalled because of its potential to cause greater risk of heart attacks and strokes—illustrating how broad the effects of a drug targeted to treat one problem can actually be.

The natural alternatives are generally much safer than most pharmaceutical options. To learn about natural alternatives to the NSAIDS, read *Pain Free in 6 Weeks* by Sherry Rogers, MD, and *Natural Alternatives to Vioxx, Celebrex, and Other Anti-Inflammatory Drugs* by Carol Simontacchi, MS, CCN. However, it is possible to overdo even natural substances. There is a rule in toxicology: "The dose makes the poison." Almost anything overdone can become a problem. I once managed to give myself heartburn from daily consumption of a very strong extract made from ginger root, a natural anti-inflammatory. I now use a more moderate amount of this otherwise wonderful herb and have experienced no further problems.

Don't Remain Constipated

Many people experience both constipation and heartburn. Constipation can be caused by as well as contribute to faulty digestion. Regularity pays off with less digestive stress and less heartburn. Laxatives, however, have side effects, and I don't recommend them as a heartburn remedy. Instead, since constipation and heartburn are aggravated by the same things—such as insufficient water, low fiber dietary choices, low stomach acid, stress, and imbalances in GI microbes (like insufficient good bacteria and yeast overgrowth)—it is wise to adopt healthful habits that will benefit both.

Lose Weight

Research has found a connection between acid reflux and obesity. Being overweight is thought to put physical pressure on the stomach, and there is scientific evidence that losing weight does reduce symptoms of acid relux.[5] The association, however, may not always be cause and effect. Rather, the connection is likely to be the factors that cause both problems. These factors include eating fast, eating large meals, eating too late at night, eating foods to which you are sensitive or that feed yeast, eating too many refined carbohydrates (comfort and snack foods), having insufficient stomach acid, and drinking excess alcohol. If you are overweight, there are many health and quality of life reasons to address these habits. Although the weight loss may take a bit of time, you are likely to see improvement in your heartburn almost instantly.

Nutritionist Liz Lipski said, "The word 'diet' comes from Greek and means 'a manner of living' or 'way of life.'" The best diets are those that are adopted without the dieter feeling deprived. Dieters on easily managed and satisfying smart-carbohydrate diets often lose pounds quickly, while also enjoying prompt relief of heartburn and symptoms like sleep apnea and Candida overgrowth. Dr. Fred Pescatore has written *The Hamptons Diet*, a guide to healthful delicious meal plans that limit carbs. He states, "The Hamptons Diet eliminates the foods that lead to inflammation, which is a major cause of acid reflux. If you eliminate the offending foods, the reflux and the associated health risks will disappear without the use of potentially harmful medications."

There may be other digestive issues affecting your ability to lose weight. For example, readjusting stomach acid and enzymes so that they are present in the proper levels can help with weight loss because if you are not digesting and absorbing the nutrients in your meals, you will be hungry all the time. An under-active thyroid can cause unhealthy weight gain and then make it difficult to lose weight. To determine if that might be an issue, take the thyroid quiz on my website, www.RadioMartie.com.

Resolve Other Health Issues

Any condition that puts pressure on the stomach can be an issue. For instance, constant coughing can force stomach contents upstream. (It is worth noting that a lingering cough that stumps doctors may be caused by yeast.) Pregnancy, too, can cause acid reflux. Of course, full resolution of this particular trigger typically takes about nine months. Because of the unknown effects of acid blockers on the fetus, pregnancy may be a great time to explore the natural remedies.

CONCLUSION

Although many doctors of conventional medicine may be quick to point acid-reflux sufferers toward a solution like surgery or pharmaceutical medications, there are many other options available. Some of these effective alternatives, many of which were covered in this chapter, may even offer fringe benefits instead of side effects. The next chapter will look at probiotics and the important role they play in your health.

CHAPTER 10

CARE AND FEEDING
OF THE GOOD BUGS

"Gold that buys health can never be ill spent."
—THOMAS DEKKER

Dietary supplements can be an important tool in resolving all kinds of gastrointestinal distress. However, they help us obtain the best results when we do not used them as though they were drugs: we limit benefit if we consider natural supplements as simply benign silver bullets used to suppress our symptoms. Although they are safer than pharmaceuticals, you are best off utilizing supplements to solve the root problem rather than simply alleviate symptoms. Also, to provide the most long-term benefits, supplements should be used in conjunction with diet and lifestyle changes. This chapter will discuss probiotics, which are available as supplements that make fundamental contributions with far-reaching benefits. Supplements that are focused on symptom relief and damage repair will be described in Chapter 11.

Most American consumers spend money on nonessentials—from gourmet coffee to magazines and from fads to cigarettes—every single day. Those small purchases add up substantially. Yet many of these same people are unwilling to invest even a modest amount in high quality dietary supplements that might save or at least improve their lives! Probiotics and other supplements can be as, if not more, effective than medications in many cases, and deserve a higher spot on most consumers' lists of priorities.

THE BENEFITS OF PROBIOTICS

Good bacteria are called *probiotics*, which means "for life." Everyone—all living creatures—must have them to live. Bacteria—of which the human body contains three to four pounds—are located throughout the body, but the majority is found in the digestive tract. It has recently come to light that the much-dismissed and often-removed appendix acts as a back-up storage compartment for probiotics. If the main supply is wiped out by something like dysentery, the appendix is in charge of repopulating the colon.

Unfortunately, we sometimes make life tough for our good bacteria. *Antibiotics* are substances that kill bacteria. The word literally means "against life." Antibiotics can certainly be life saving if taken appropriately and when necessary, but they tend to kill all the bacteria—the good and the bad—with which they come into contact. To understand how this can affect our health, let's take a look at the positive role that probiotics have on our bodies.

Protection from Harmful Bacteria

As we established in Chapter 4, stomach acid is our first line of defense against disease-causing bacteria. Our friendly bacteria are crucial defenders as well. Probiotics compete with the negative bacteria for both food and space. They also create chemicals, such as bacteriocins, that wipe out pathogens like *H. pylori*. Some of the bacteria that they can be effective against are among the most troubling: Salmonella, *E. Coli, C. Difficile*, and Methicillin-resistant *Staphylococcus aureus* (MRSA). (MRSA is an especially treacherous bacterium that annually sickens 90,000 people—and kills thousands—in the United States alone.) Today, many strains of disease-causing bacteria have become resistant to antibiotics and cannot be treated with our old standby medicines, so it is increasingly important to have your natural defenses in full force.

Balance of Parasites and Yeast

Stomach acid is not only the first line of defense against bacteria, but also parasites and yeast. But these invaders do sometimes make it past the hydrochloric acid—especially if a person is taking an acid blocker. The good news is that a digestive system that is properly stocked with protective bacteria can help protect the body against unhealthy bacteria and fungus that slip past the stomach.

Increased Number of Immune Cells

Most of our immune system can be found along our intestinal tract. Probiotics help us produce immune cells by maintaining the health of our intestinal lining. Immune cells go after and destroy disease-producing organisms as well as cancerous tissue, which has been damaged or is reproducing abnormally.

Assistance with Digestion

Probiotics play an important role in the digestion of many food products. These organisms, for example, break down cellulose, a plant fiber. We need this help because humans don't make an enzyme for that purpose. Probiotics also help break down lactose—milk sugar—and a large percentage of the population cannot digest it on its own because of a lack of the enzyme lactase. Probiotics also indirectly assist our bodies in the production of stomach acid and digestive enzymes, because those processes are supported by the ability of our digestive tract to extract the needed raw materials from our food.

Detoxification of Harmful Substances

Probiotics process cancer-causing chemicals into more stable substances, which can then be escorted out of the body. They also help keep excess estrogen from being reabsorbed into circulation, which protects against hormone-dependent cancers like breast cancer and perhaps prostate cancer.

Free radicals, or oxidants, are unstable molecules that damage parts of our cells. Depending on what part of the body they damage, these molecules can cause heart disease or cancer. Antioxidants are delivered in foods and supplements, and help protect the body from this damage. Probiotics, especially when along with their food, called *prebiotics*, improve our body's antioxidant status.

Production of Vitamins

The beneficial bacteria are involved in making vitamins A, B_1, B_2, B_3, B_6, B_{12}, K, and biotin. The production of these vitamins is very important for good health.

It is particularly beneficial to have this internal source of vitamin A because vegetable foods don't provide this vitamin directly. Instead, they provide carotene, which the body—with the help of both probiotics and enzymes—can then make into vitamin A. Vitamin A is especially helpful to the health of mucus membranes, like those that line the digestive tract and lungs. A lack of vitamin A may cause the esophagus and stomach to be unable to effectively repair themselves.

Vitamin K may not be frequently discussed, but is important as well. It helps keep calcium out of the lining of the arteries and helps it into bones and muscle cells. This allows the body to perform work such as closing the LES.

Health of the Intestinal Tract Lining

Probiotics digest fiber so that it releases essential fatty acids, which, in turn, feed the gut lining. As discussed in Chapter 7, an unhealthy intestinal lining can lead to allergies, autoimmune disorders, and other health conditions. Friendly flora also help reduce populations of unhealthful organisms, such as yeast, that might otherwise damage the intestinal lining.

Maintenance of Healthy Cholesterol Levels

Consumers have been told to cut down on foods that contain cholesterol. However, the majority of circulating cholesterol is made in the body. One reason for a buildup of cholesterol in arteries is that the excess is supposed to be taken care of in the intestinal tract and expelled, but this can be hindered if the tract is not healthy.

Another cause of cholesterol excess can be generalized inflammation. Unfortunately, the standard treatment for elevated cholesterol does not look at the status of the digestive tract or the cause of the inflammation. Instead, most doctors prescribe statin drugs to force the cholesterol down at the risk of many potentially serious side effects, including heartburn. Probiotics, on the other hand, can help you maintain healthy cholesterol and triglyceride levels while providing you with fringe benefits as opposed to potentially negative side effects.[1] *The Cholesterol Hoax* by Sherry Rogers, MD, is a good source of natural answers to the cholesterol question.

Reduction of Inflammation

The inflammatory response is a natural process of the body to injury and infection. However, inflammation can also become chronic and cause gastritis, heart disease, and joint problems. It may be true that statin drugs have an anti-inflammatory aspect, but probiotics are one of many safer approaches to reducing inflammation. (Other options are discussed on pages 183 to 184.)

Aging More Slowly

There are two ways to determine peoples' ages: by their calendar age and by their much more important *functional age*. It is this second measurement—which is evaluated based on the relative condition of the body and its ability to function properly—that probiotics can improve. They help all systems work better, while also working to limit the absorption of toxins and foreign particles into circulation. They also stimulate cell repair mechanisms and greatly increase what are thought of as anti-aging detoxifying antioxidant enzymes.

Improvement of Mood

Believe it or not, probiotics can help you be happier. This may seem far-fetched, but up to 90 percent of your body's serotonin receptors and much of its production are located in the gut. Serotonin is a neurotransmitter with many responsibilities, including the regulation of your mood. It is often referred to as

---

Friendly Yeast

Just as there are bacteria that are good for you, there are also yeasts with health benefits. *Saccharomyces boulardii* (SB) is a type of yeast that acts as a probiotic. It steps up the production of enzymes and stimulates the immune system in the intestinal mucosa. Although it is transient and should not be used to replace probiotics, some people see benefits from supplementing SB, especially while on an antibiotic. That is because SB is resistant to commonly used antibiotics and helps keep bad yeasts under control during treatment. Anti-fungals would harm these yeasts, as they do all yeasts. I recommend products by Florastor and Jarrow Formulas.

the "happy hormone." When our bacteria are out of balance and especially when yeasts take over, depression, anxiety, and even aggression can emerge. On the other hand, when the intestines are balanced, we feel good and are even inclined to eat more healthful food.

The balance of organisms in the digestive tract always falls on a continuum somewhere between all good and all bad guys. We never totally eliminate the bad guys, and that's okay. However, it becomes a problem when they could get very out of hand—which can happen quite quickly since bacteria can double their numbers every thirty minutes. Unless we are providing the right environment for the good guys, we can develop big problems as the disease fostering strains flourish.

The technical term for an imbalance of digestive organisms is *dysbiosis*. Symptoms of this deteriorating situation in your digestive tract may begin subtly and can be easy to miss for some time. (See page 97 for a list of possible symptoms.)

STRENGTHENING YOUR SUPPLY OF PROBIOTICS

It should be clear that protecting your probiotics must be a high priority. Much of what was described in Chapter 7 regarding keeping yeasts from getting out of control are steps that will also preserve our colonies of good bacteria. These actions include avoiding unnecessary antibiotics, improving the diet (especially by eliminating sugar, other sweet things, and white flour), and reducing stress and toxic exposure. However, even if you studiously avoid these damaging factors, modern life is just hard on the good guys in our digestive tract, so nearly everyone can benefit from supplementing probiotics.

Food Sources

The people of many cultures routinely eat fermented foods, which provide replenishment of friendly bacteria. Asians, for example, usually consume traditionally brewed soy sauce or tamari. Yet in the United States, these same products are often made with chemicals instead of through bacterial fermentation. Likewise, sauerkraut in Eastern Europe contains active cultures, but the US-required pasteurization kills the bacteria. The most common fermented food eaten in the United States is yogurt. Unfortunately, there are problems with depending on this source for probiotics: dairy allergy is common, the number of strains used is limited, and the bacterial cultures may no longer be alive and/or are not types to remain in the gut. The most popular yogurt products also contain high amounts of sugar which, besides being inflammatory, feed yeasts and reduce immune function.

Probiotic Supplements

Most probiotic supplements, even the simpler and less potent ones, do at least some good, but certain types of products are just plain superior to others. There is also one type that I believe requires caution. It pays to be an educated consumer.

Freeze-Dried Cultures

Freeze-dried cultures, like all probiotics, are best when they contain a variety of strains, because each strain serves different functions. Supplementing large amounts of just one, two, or three strains can upset the balance, send an alarm signal to the immune system, and potentially even trigger an autoimmune response. When dealing with these products, be aware that your body may have a hard time waking the critters from their freeze-dried coma because the cells may have been damaged by the processes of drying and centrifuging, which spins the culture to separate the bacteria from the culture medium.

In products of this type, the various strains are combined after they are dried to keep them from competing with and killing each other. However, when they hit the digestive tract, it is every bug for itself as they try to stake out their territory. This type of product usually uses dairy or soy, which can be allergenic, as a base for growing the organisms. The centrifuging separates the organisms from that base, which somewhat reduces the allergic potential, but also leaves the bugs without the food supply to which they are accustomed. Centrifuging also breaks up the colonies into individual cells, which are more fragile.

Freeze-dried products typically require refrigeration at the store and at home because they are not stable at room temperature. I haven't seen studies on the stability of the refrigerated dry types once opened in the home, but it stands to reason that they are a little less dry each time you open the bottle and room humidity condenses on the capsules or powder. I prefer live bacteria to the dried type, but Jarro-Dophilus is one freeze-dried product that I think is above average. It contains six strains of probiotics and is prepared using high standards.

Soil-Based Organisms

Many different types of bacteria are found in soil. Some of them may have benefit, but some will kill us. That is one reason we usually do not eat dirt. Yet one soil-based probiotic, supplied by a multi-level company, was developed in a responsible way and can be beneficial to our health. Although its strain was originally isolated from soil, it has been carefully stabilized in a laboratory for thousands of bacterial generations. That product has held up to the test of time. Unfortunately, there are other soil-based products that have not. One retail product that popularized the idea of soil-based organisms and made its developer quite wealthy was not so carefully researched for safety and benefit of the strains. A great many practitioners have reported that it caused severe long-lasting digestive distress. I found that my clients who tried it had a few days of feeling good, followed by a development of digestive issues. Make sure to read a company's research before buying this type of probiotic product. You can also do an internet search for both consumer and professional reviews to gather more information.

Live Organisms in a Biogenic Matrix

The newest type of probiotics product delivers the beneficial bacteria alive. This eliminates worry about whether the probiotics will wake up after being freeze-dried. Culturing the various strains together means that there is also less concern about territorial competition. It further ensures viability if the probiotics are encapsulated with their own accustomed food supply. I recommend finding a product that also contains the substances produced naturally during fermentation. These include those bacteriocins (discussed on page 170) that help control pathogenic bacteria. Probiotics also produce organic acids, which improve the environment of the digestive tract and therefore the lives of all our hundreds of probiotic strains. This is very important because each of us has a unique blend of friendly bacteria and we cannot possibly supplement them all.

My favorite product—which, as far as I know, is the only one available that meets all these criteria—is Dr. Ohhira's Probiotic 12 Plus. It is fermented at room temperature so that it doesn't need refrigeration. It is also vegan, including the capsule. (See Resources section for information on where this product can be purchased.) For routine use, take this supplement every day. Take two capsules a day, preferably in two separate doses. I advise my clients to wait until their stomach has emptied or at least calmed down, approximately one to one-and-a-half hours after a meal. Others recommend taking these supplements on a totally empty stomach first thing in the morning. If you are not in a delicate state of health and want faster results, you can take five capsules twice a day for the first six days. I have seen no evidence that it is possible to overdose on this safe and balanced product. In the next chapter, I will talk about chewing a couple of capsules after a meal for instant relief of acid indigestion symptoms.

KEEPING YOUR PROBIOTICS WELL FED

Just like people, gut bacteria are quite sensitive to their food supply. For example, if you usually eat a high protein/low carbohydrate diet and go on a vegetarian kick with lots of grains and fruits, your friendly bugs will need to become accustomed to this whole new diet. Some bacteria that were acclimated to the old diet will die down while those that can subsist on the new diet take hold and multiply. There can be symptoms of gas or a change in bowel function during the transition.

Fiber is important because certain kinds allow probiotics to flourish. There are three kinds of fiber: *insoluble fiber*, which is not broken down in the intestines and is sometimes referred to as "roughage"; *soluble fiber*, which helps lower cholesterol and is found in oatmeal, fruits, beans, and some vegetables such as broccoli; and *resistant starch*, which is found naturally in unripe bananas, whole grains, lentils, and beans. Soluble fiber is good because probiotics thrive on it while pathogenic bacteria do not. The good guys also like resistant starch.

Prebiotics are foods purposely supplemented to promote the growth of good bacteria. If you are not taking the type of probiotic system that comes with its own food supply or if you simply want to encourage the further growth of your own friendly strains, you may want to consider a prebiotic. Some products used for the purpose are inulin and fructooligosaccharides (FOS). They are extracted from fruits and vegetables. However, be careful not to overdo consumption of these

The Prebiotic Arabinogalactan

Arabinogalactan is a complex carbohydrate extracted from the timber of a larch tree and consumed to encourage the health and growth of probiotics. It is found in a product called FiberAid, which is produced by the company Lonza. I recommend this product to my clients and listeners of my radio show because it is extracted from the tree using a process without chemicals. Although it has been shown to be safe up to 30 grams a day, I have found that 4.5 grams a day is very effective. It is not a significant source of calories and has no glycemic effect, making it fine for use by diabetics. Arabinogalactan is available as FiberAid, a powder with little taste, and as a tablet from Jarrow under the name Larix 1000.

Arabinogalactan supplementation can have quite a few positive effects on your health. These include the following:

- It helps friendly bacteria grow and multiply.

- It reduces levels of the unfriendly bacteria Clostridium and *E. Coli*.

- By feeding the probiotics, it indirectly increases the function of short chain fatty acids (SCFAs), which in turn provide a major source of energy for the cells that line the intestinal tract. One SCFA in particular, Butyrate, provides about half the fuel for the gastrointestinal cells.[2] Short chain fatty acids also provide energy to the brain, muscle, and heart and may protect colon cells from tumors.

- It decreases the intestine's manufacture and absorption of ammonia—a substance that is not good for the intestinal cells. In excess, ammonia can cause confusion and even coma.

- It may have some antiviral properties, as exhibited in some animals studies.

products. They are known to cause gas and bloating. Additionally, it is of some concern that a number of unfriendly strains of bugs seem to be keen on FOS if it is present in too great a supply.

I recommend arabinogalactan (an extract from a tree) in a product called FiberAid by Lonza. It ferments slowly, so is well tolerated, and has been shown in studies to be beneficial in several ways. See the inset on page 180 for a list of benefits that arabinogalactan provide.

CONCLUSION

If you support your friendly colonies, they will support you. Over time, especially in conjunction with an improved diet, supplementing and supporting your probiotics will provide you with greatly improved digestion and better overall health because of the fundamental role they play. Our health is a team effort, and probiotics play a big part. The next chapter will focus on other natural supplements, which can be used for repair of certain health problems or relief from symptoms.

CHAPTER 11

SUPPLEMENTS FOR RELIEF AND REPAIR

"Adam and Eve ate the first vitamins, including the package."
—E. R. SQUIBB

There are many useful natural supplements for people suffering from acid reflux. Some deal with the initial cause of the problem, others restore damaged tissue, and still others provide symptom relief. Chapter 10 described those supplements that deal with the root cause. This chapter will be divided into two parts. First, we will discuss supplements that can be utilized to treat the damage caused by the heartburn and ulcers, and to help reduce inflammation. (Please note that DGL is listed in this first group but also brings symptomatic relief.) The second half of the chapter will describe supplements that can help relieve symptoms. Taking these supplements and making the diet and lifestyle changes we've discussed may allow you to see immediate relief, but that is no substitute for diagnosing and treating the underlying cause—which may include a hiatus hernia, low stomach acid, and/or overgrowth of *H. pylori* or Candida.

Don't let the number of remedies discourage you. You may not even need any of them after trying some of the changes in the previous chapters. However, as you read through, you are likely to find one that best describes your situation, and you can start supplementation with that product. Trial and error is also an option because these supplements are generally safe.

You should always discuss your treatment plan with your doctor. If your heartburn is caused by a bleeding ulceration, for example, your doctor may quite reasonably suggest that you temporarily go on an acid-blocking medication. Also, if you have had frequent and long-standing heartburn, finding relief from the symptoms may not be so easy, and your physician may be able to help. If you have an open-minded doctor, allow him or her to read this book and then help you explore the options described.

HEALING THE IRRITATED MEMBRANES

The body is amazingly resilient. Most tissues repair themselves on a scheduled basis, by getting rid of damaged cells and replacing them anew. In less than a week, you can grow new *villi*—little fingers in the intestines that help the body absorb nutrients. If the conditions are right (meaning you have stopped annoying the tissues and have rebalanced the friendly organisms), you may have all new cells up and down your gut within a month.

Healing is something the body does naturally. However, there are ways in which we can assist this process. This section will look at natural products that can help our body heal more effectively. Natural substances similar to what the body is used to producing and processing are usually healthier choices than synthetically derived chemicals.

Although healing is a natural body process, it cannot start effectively until you stop doing whatever originally caused the injury. Please keep in mind that if you are taking a non-steroidal anti-inflammatory drug (NSAID), including aspirin, you will have an uphill battle healing ulcers and irritations because the drugs are often quite damaging to the same tissues you are attempting to heal.[1] According to Dr. Georges

Halpern, one in four people who regularly take these drugs develops an ulcer. If you are on such a medication, request an alternative to a COX-1 or COX-2 inhibitor. Unfortunately, though, these drugs can have cardiovascular side effects. If you simply must take an NSAID, then supplement with Zinc-Carnosine (see page 185) because it is shown to limit the damage to the stomach lining from the likes of aspirin.[2] Also, until you are healed, you will probably want to ease up on any food or beverage that creates a burning sensation as it goes down.

The following natural substances have been researched thoroughly and found to be successful for many cases of heartburn. I have started with the products I have found most likely to work for typical acid reflux. The specifics of your case and your preferences will impact which supplement or combination of supplements works for you. Other substances that have shown some promise are the flavonoid quercetin, Japanese Panax ginseng, guar gum, myrrh gum, and capsicum (red chili pepper).[3]

DGL

Deglycyrrhizinated licorice (DGL) is an herbal supplement that can be extremely useful in healing stomach issues. Real licorice contains glycyrrhizin, a substance that is worrisome because it can cause problems like water retention and high blood pressure. However, the invention of a process that removes most of the glycyrrhizin from licorice has made DGL practical to use.

DGL heals and protects stomach tissues by increasing the sturdiness and effectiveness of the lining of the GI tract. It has nearly the same rate of success in healing ulcers as the acid-blocking drugs. (I'd love to see a study combining this with the Zinc-Carnosine covered below.)

In *Encyclopedia of Nutritional Supplements,* Dr. Michael Murray recommends DGL for healing of canker sores (ulcers in the mouth) and stomach ulcers, so it surely works on the areas in between those two parts, such as in the esophagus. In *Why Stomach Acid is Good for You*, Dr. Jonathan V. Wright recommends chewing two tablets three to four times a day, an hour before meals, and chasing with a very small amount of water. He says his patients report getting as much or more relief with regular use of DGL as with antacids or acid blockers—and without the side effects.

As for fringe benefits, there is evidence that DGL may help with food sensitivity. It also has some antibacterial effects which would theoretically be useful if a person had *H. pylori*. In a study on a combination drug approach to *H. pylori*, the DGL's theorized antibacterial effect didn't speed the eradication of the bug but did reduce the relapse rate.[4, 5, 6, 7] The folklore on licorice suggests many other benefits but they have not been well documented. I recommend trying that of the Natural Factors brand or the one from Enzymatic Therapy.

Please note that most licorice candies do not contain real licorice. They do not provide any health benefits, and contain high amounts of sugar and starch.

Zinc-Carnosine

Support for the GI tract's natural defenses should include Zinc-Carnosine, a dietary supplement that is a patented complex of the mineral zinc with the amino acid carnosine. Carnosine is found naturally in muscle and brain. Zinc-Carnosine has been shown to adhere to the damaged areas in the intestinal tract and synergistically form a protective barrier against stomach acid. This combination works better than the components do when working separately.[8, 9] Thankfully, Zinc-Carnosine does not reduce stomach acid and therefore does not interfere with digestion. It also exerts a powerful anti-inflammatory effect on the membranes and provides significant antioxidant protection for the cells.[2, 10] It is best known for healing ulcers. It also assists in the treatment of *H. pylori*. Zinc-Carnosine can help prevent GI irritation and slow the formation of stomach ulcerations, including those caused by *H. pylori* and NSAIDs.[2, 11] It is possible that thousands of lives would be saved if everyone on an NSAID painkiller was advised to also take Zinc-Carnosine, which has been found to be a very safe natural remedy. As with many drugs and supplements, though, tests have not been performed on children or pregnant women.

Most studies of this product have been in relation to stomach problems, but there is evidence that it may also improve esophageal heartburn. Therefore, Zinc-Carnosine is a particularly useful supplement because often people can't tell if their pain originates in their esophagus or stomach (or both). Fringe benefits of this supplement include positive effects for people suffering from nausea, vomiting, bloating, and anorexia.

Besides the synergy of zinc in combination with carnosine over the use of either component separately, I prefer this form of zinc over other types because it seems to act more locally and is less likely to overload the system and cause mineral imbalances. As Dr. Halpern suggests in *Ulcer Free!*, take 75.5 milligrams with food twice a day for eight weeks. I recommend PepZinGI by Jarrow.

Colostrum

Colostrum may be the most comprehensive and powerful natural supplement. The initial fluid from the mother's breast when mammals give birth, colostrum is a rich and complex blend of almost miraculous immune and growth factors. It provides the newborn with the ability to begin maturing various bodily systems.

One action of colostrum is to discourage the attachment of pathogenic bacteria to the mucosal lining.[12] Athletes revere colostrum because it helps with tissue healing and recovery. The healing action of colostrum can be observed when used topically on skin irritations and wounds. The mucus membranes are the skin of our insides, so it is logical that calming of the irritation and damage associated with heartburn is one of the potential benefits, although research that specific is scant. The immune modulation it provides will also help with any infection that might be part of the problem[13] as well as many other aspects of health, because the immune system is crucially important to nearly every part of life, possibly even including weight. Another relevant positive effect of colostrum is that it improves the viability of probiotics.[14] Fringe benefits include help with blood sugar management, cholesterol, liver health, and allergies. It is also a powerful booster of detoxifying enzymes. One such enzyme, glutathione peroxidase, is a key to neutralizing free radicals that attack tissues. A study showed that potent colostrum increased glutathione by as much as 100 percent in two hours. According to Richard Cockrum, DVM, who has spent over forty years researching the material, "colostrum can help in so many disparate ways because it is a complex of many beneficial substances that work at a very basic cellular level."

Colostrum for supplementation is obtained from cows. The quality and potency of the supplement is quite important. You want to take 100-percent true colostrum, which can only be obtained in the first six hours after birth. The second milking liquid contains only 16-percent colostrum, with the balance being milk. Therefore, look for colostrum labeled as "First Collection Colostrum." Donor cows that provide the richest concentration of immune and growth factors must be mature—aged three years or older—as well as exceptionally well nourished and provided with superior prenatal care. Another crucial factor is that the natural balance should not be corrupted with laboratory manipulations after harvesting and there should not be any residues of antibiotics, added hormones, or pesticides. PerCoBa meets all these requirements— and buying this product supports small American family dairy farms that have a Grade A rating.

Fish Oil

Fish oil has many important effects on health, due in large part to its being a rich source of omega-3 fatty acids. Among the benefits are its actions as an anti-inflammatory. This function is particularly useful for those with inflammation of the GI tract, as is the case with heartburn, gastritis, ulcers, and so forth. Recent British research suggested that continued supplementation with EPA, a constituent of fish oil, caused improvement in the cells of the mucous membranes of the esophagus in subjects diagnosed with Barrett's Esophagus—a condition caused by acid reflux and a precursor to esophageal cancer in 10 percent of sufferers.[15] Fish oil is also known, among other effects, to promote heart-health, to protect against several cancers, and to relieve joint pain and even depression.

Many "experts" and various media are quick to call any supplement with claims of multiple benefits "snake oil." They aim to insult the product with comparison to oil of snake products sold by old-time traveling patent medicine merchants. Although consumers often reported benefit, those products were accused of being no more than marketing hype and ultimately fell out of favor when drugs and organized medicine came on the scene. In contrast, the positive science on omega-3 fats is so extensive that, in spite of the broad range of benefits experienced with fish oil, both the medical and media fields have been supportive. Yet snake oil is exceptionally high in omega-3 fats—leading me to hypothesize that those old travel-ing medicine men may have had something worthwhile after all! (Snake oil is still sold for pain relief in traditional pharma-cies, but not often in western countries.)

Although flax oil can also be a good source of omega-3 fatty acids, it does not include DHA or EPA—the heralded con-stituents of fish oil—and so should not be relied upon as the sole source of omega-3, except for strict vegetarians. Unfortu-nately, even eating a lot of fish does not necessarily provide you with enough essential fatty acids because farmed fish usu-ally have less omega-3 than wild fish contain. There is also concern regarding mercury contamination of many fish sources. For these reasons, I suggest supplementing your omega-3 intake with fish oil supplements.

The key factors in selecting a fish oil supplement are fresh-ness and assurance that the oil does not contain mercury or other heavy metals. Nordic Naturals excels in those standards and is available in most natural food stores. The liquids are the best value and taste much better than you might expect. Nordic has high potency capsules as well.

Combination Products

The professional brand Biotics Research offers a product called BIO-HPF. It combines deglycyrrhizinated licorice (DGL; described on pages 184 to 185), slippery elm bark, berberine, bismuth citrate, myrrh, clove, and anise powder. The formula is designed to control *H. pylori*, reduce inflammation, and heal tissue. It is available from many nutritionists, chiropractors, and compounding pharmacies.

Reflux-Away from NaturalCare combines several homeo-pathic remedies with unspecified amounts of HCl, DGL, gin-ger, mastic, and other items, and is available in health food stores. It may bring you symptom relief, and also has healing

ingredients. There is information on other homeopathic remedies on page 203.

Vitamins and Minerals

The nutrients described in this section are essential for many
functions other than digestive health. Also, more nutrients
than are described here are required by your body in order to
properly heal. Therefore, although supplementation can help
and is quite important, there is no substitute for a varied diet of
nutrient-dense food.

A Multi-Vitamin and Mineral

Although doctors used to think a so-called balanced diet provided all necessary nutrition, it is now generally agreed that
this type of supplement is a modern-day necessity because of
mineral-depleted soils, processed foods, and our increased
need generated by exposure to toxins in the environment. Start
with a broad professionally balanced base that fills in the gaps
from your diet and avoids excess. You are better off getting a
multi from a health food store than buying one of the discount
store brands or one that is highly advertised. The big mass market names can afford all that advertising because they skimp
on the expensive ingredients and the more costly but better
absorbed delivery forms. There are many excellent choices.
With a multi as a base, you can add additional amounts of
some of the following—but be aware of the amount in the
multi and be careful not to overload on any particular one.

Calcium

Calcium helps strengthen the LES. Counterproductively, acid
blockers inhibit the absorption of calcium. Because calcium is
bulky, most multi-vitamins contain only a small amount, so a
separate supplement is often advisable. Clearly, as you read in

Chapter 3, calcium-based antacids are usually not a good solution to the problem of acid reflux. Fortunately, there are other types available.

For regular use and bone health, I recommend finding an absorbable and balanced form such as BoneUp by Jarrow because it contains a highly useable form of calcium (microcrystalline hydroxyapatite) plus a number of other minerals and nutrients to assure proper utilization. Dr. Leo Galland offers another approach: he recommends 250 milligrams of calcium citrate powder, dissolved in water, after every meal and at bedtime (for a total daily dose of 1,000 milligrams) to solve the problem of a lazy LES. Do not combine this regimen with BoneUp. Too much calcium, especially if not balanced with magnesium and other minerals, can cause constipation and other issues.

Vitamin D

Vitamin D is needed for immune function (including protection against *H. pylori*) and muscle strength such as that needed to close the LES,[16] but levels of this important vitamin are lowered by some medications such as prednisone and methotrexate. People report more heartburn in the winter. The seasonality of this complaint may be partly because our bodies make vitamin D when our skin is exposed to the sun, and we tend to get less exposure in the winter. Perhaps another indirect reason is that we eat fewer of the fruits and vegetables that help us absorb vitamin D during the winter. Attaining normal vitamin D levels requires twenty minutes of sunshine a day without sunscreen and with some substantial part of your skin exposed, or consumption of a vitamin D_3 (cholecalciferol) supplement. The government recommends a dose of 2,000 IU per day as an upper limit. That is safe for most people. Many people take more than this under professional supervision. Only a few individuals have a hypersensitivity.

Vitamin C

Vitamin C has many responsibilities. It helps reduce inflammation in the digestive tract. It is associated with decreases in *H. pylori* infections and even inhibits stomach cancer growth. It also helps heal gastritis.[17, 18] Studies usually show that the most beneficial vitamin C is that acquired directly from food. This is most likely due in part to the presence of a vitamin C partner, bioflavanoids. If you are going to take vitamin C supplements, you need to be aware of the different types. Ascorbic acid, vitamin C in its simplest supplemental form, is acidic. However, in the form of mineral ascorbates, that acidity is buffered. As a bonus, the ascorbates also contain needed minerals.

Vitamin E

Vitamin E has been popular for a long time because of its cardiovascular benefits. More recently, animal studies have shown vitamin E to be protective of the stomach and speed the healing of stomach lesions.[19] It has also been shown to help inflammatory conditions such as allergies, asthma,[20] heartburn, and gastritis.

It is quite important to use the natural (*d-alpha*) form of vitamin E rather than the synthetic (*dl-alpha*). The synthetic versions are not nearly as effective. Likewise, much better results are attained from using the entire E complex, which includes gamma-tocopherol and its family members, as opposed to the most common supplemental forms, which contain only d-alpha. This is for two reasons. One, gamma-tocopherol is quite potent in its own right. Two, supplementing one member of a nutrient group may create an artificial shortage of the other members because of competition for absorption routes.

Zinc

There are many important reasons, such as proper immune function and healing ulcerations,[11] to assure that our bodies absorb sufficient amounts of zinc. As you read in Chapter 4, stomach acid is necessary for this absorption. At the same time, if the stomach lining is not healthy because of a zinc or other nutrient deficiency, we cannot create stomach acid. This is, therefore, another one of those potentially vicious cyles. If you are in that situation, you should supplement both zinc and acid.

Vitamin A

Vitamin A is important to the health of mucous membranes, and may reduce the size of ulcers.[21] It also aids the immune system. Carrots are commonly thought to be a great source of vitamin A, but they do not actually contain this vitamin. Rather, carrots contain carotenes, which your body can then turn into vitamin A, provided that all the necessary bodily systems are working properly. Probiotics make vitamin A as well.

Supplements labeled "vitamin A" as opposed to "carotene" will provide faster results. However, you can certainly take both. If you do choose to take a carotene supplement in addition to your vitamin A supplement, buy a product—which can be either oil or dry—that contains the entire natural carotene complex, rather than just the popular beta-carotene, so as not to cause an imbalance.

Magnesium

Magnesium is used in hundreds of enzyme reactions. It is important to prevent spasms of muscles and sphincters and to promote regularity of bowel movements—which is particularly noteworthy because constipation is considered a risk factor for heartburn. Magnesium oxide is cheap and readily available, but may go beyond simply correcting the problem of constipation and cause a loose stool. I prefer a more absorbable form such as a magnesium chelate, and recommend those produced by Albion Labs.

Aloe Vera

A desert plant, aloe vera has an ancient reputation for improving digestion. You may have seen its healing magic work on a burn, sunburn, or wound. It has the same effect on our insides. Modern science indicates that it has an anti-inflammatory effect (even when the inflammation is caused by *H. pylori*), detoxifying properties, and the ability to help heal ulcerations. Its constituent mannose may help probiotics adhere in the intestines, while also keeping Candida yeast from doing the same.[22, 23]

There is *extremely* wide variability in the quality of aloe vera products. They should have a light vegetable flavor, and can come in either juice or gel form. Regardless of the type, the dosage remains the same: 2 to 8 ounces per day. I always recommend starting slowly with any new supplement in case you experience an allergic or other atypical reaction. I have researched and used many aloe vera products, and recommend trying Manapol or Lily of the Desert organic products. These companies protect the active ingredients from harmful processing techniques and their products contain the highest concentration of the active ingredients—polysaccharides—when compared to other brands.

Watch out for products that have a very bitter flavor and capsules that promise a laxative effect. This undesirable effect is caused when preparers do not avoid the yellow sap in the rind—and the laxative effect is harsh. On the other end of the spectrum, avoid products that taste like water because that may be all you are getting. When a product is distilled to remove flavor, its healing qualities are also removed.

Cabbage Juice/L-Glutamine

In a booklet entitled *10 Drugs I Would Never Take*, Dr. Joseph E. Pizzorno, Jr. (a founder of renown Bastyr University) discusses two studies related to the effects of L-glutamine on health. One demonstrated that one liter per day of fresh cabbage juice—which contains L-glutamine—could heal ulcers in ten days.[24] The other study tested just the amino acid. A dose of 1.6 grams per day of L-glutamine was more effective at healing ulcers than the conventional treatment, which would have included antacids and dietary modification.[25]

Cabbage juice is great for reducing pain from and healing mouth ulcers. It is likely to do the same for ulcers of the esophagus and stomach. L-glutamine is available as a supplement in powder, capsule, or tablet form. One study illustrated the effects of L-glutamine in supporting the intestinal membranes of rats receiving radiation treatment on their abdomens. The results were that 100 percent of the rats survived, compared with a 45-percent survival rate among rats given a different amino acid. (Radiation is surely much worse than anything you've done to your gut with bad diet and medicines!) L-glutamine also helps increase production of glutathione, a very important detoxifying antioxidant enzyme discussed on page 187.[26]

Phosphatidylcholine

Research in Sweden concluded that supplemental phosphatidylcholine in acute cases "reduces lesions [erosions] in a dose-dependent manner and contributes to the mucosal defense."[27] *H. pylori* reduces the amount of phosphatidylcholine in the stomach. Therefore, if you are host to this bacteria, you may want to supplement phosphatidylcholine during treatment and even after the bacteria are under control.[28]

Phosphatidylcholine also has fringe benefits. The Physicians Desk Reference *Health* says, "[It] is found in soy lecithin. It can be taken as dietary lecithin or as a supplement for high cholesterol, atherosclerosis (fat deposits on arteries), high blood pressure, liver problems, bipolar depression, dementia, dyskinesias (difficulty making movements), gallbladder disease, headache, and multiple sclerosis. It is used on the skin for acne and psoriasis."

Propolis

Bees make, along with the more commonly known honey and bee pollen, a substance called propolis. It is produced from plant resins that they collect and serves as a sealant for the hive, but is also useful for protection from infection. The folklore health uses for propolis are substantial and scientific studies seem to be validating the claims one by one. Of interest here is the ability of propolis to help heal ulcers, particularly those caused by alcohol and NSAIDs.[29] This effect may come from its antibacterial, anti-fungal, anti-inflammatory, and antioxidant properties. Some potential anti-tumor activity is a welcome fringe benefit.[30] Because propolis contains as many as 300 constituents and varies depending on the originating locale, effectiveness varies greatly from product to product.[31] Brazilian green propolis is valued as highly potent and perhaps most desirable. Essential Formulas is an excellent product.

Exercise caution when utilizing propolis. Some people have an allergy to the plant sources used by the bees. Also, propolis somewhat lowered stomach secretions in an ulcer study.[29] So, unless your problem is excess acid, propolis might be best employed for short-term needs during the healing phase.

Ginkgo Biloba

Ginkgo biloba is the leaf of an ancient Asian tree. Its extract improves microcirculation all over the body and provides antioxidant protection. People typically take ginkgo as a supplement with the expectation that it will help with memory. There is some evidence that it does improve concentration and may delay dementia. In Chapter 3, I mentioned animal studies that suggest that the herb ginkgo biloba seems to help heal ulcers and reduce the pain of gastritis. Even more encouraging is evidence that it interrupts the processes that lead to gastric cancer. However, there is also at least some evidence that ginkgo may compound the blood thinning effects of medications such as aspiring and warfarin, leading to a slight risk of bleeding incidents such as stroke. Many of the substances described earlier in this chapter might be a better choice if your goal is protection and healing of the GI tract.

Testosterone

Testosterone is a powerful hormone that we all—men and women alike—need for many reasons. In his book *Why Stomach Acid Is Good for You*, Jonathan Wright, MD, suggests that "correcting unusually low levels of testosterone can help tissue repair in either sex." You must have a prescription to supplement testosterone, which, because of its power and potential for abuse, is regulated as a drug despite being a natural substance that is made by the body. Your doctor will first run tests to determine just how much testosterone is needed to bring your levels back to normal. Some mainstream doctors will prescribe patented synthetic variants of natural hormones because that is what the pharmaceutical companies promote. However, you should ask for a "bio-identical" hormone, rather than a synthetic substitute, because the body reacts differently to molecules that are not exact replicas. The bio-identical variety is available at compounding pharmacies and some mainstream pharmacies.

SYMPTOM RELIEF

The following suggestions can provide symptom relief from acid reflux. They are not alternatives to the treatments previously described in this chapter, which provide relief as well as heal the damage caused by the acid reflux. Rather, the following treatments should be used to complement the other products and provide extra relief when necessary.

Chew a Probiotic

Chapter 10 discussed probiotics as an important component of the health of the GI tract, especially the small intestine. You may also find that chewing soft gel probiotic complex capsules provides nearly immediate relief for an upset or painful stomach or after a meal. At the same time, you will also be getting all the wide-range and long-lasting benefits that come from helping improve the gut flora. The only product I know that works this way is Dr. Ohhira's Probiotics 12 Plus. Chew two or three capsules. They are safe. Because they are stable at room temperature and come in convenient blister packs, I always carry some in my purse.

General Digestive Enzymes and HCl

As discussed at length in Chapter 5, taking enzymes with meals can prevent most meal-related distress. Digestive Gold by Enzymedica is a good choice. If you suspect you are low in stomach acid, try Super Enzyme Caps by Twinlab, which contain HCl as well as enzymes. This particular supplement does not contain a lot of HCl, which is beneficial if you are experimenting as to whether your stomach acid needs to increase or decrease. If you react positively to the HCl, I recommend trying Nature's Life Betaine Hydrochloride, a pure HCl supplement, for a stronger dose. Start slowly and stop immediately if the burning gets worse instead of better.

Bitters

When low stomach acid is the cause of heartburn, bitters can help because they stimulate that phase of digestion. Begin by

A Combination Approach

A university study completed in Brazil in 2006 showed the potential of a specific combination of supplements. The amino acids L-tryptophan and L-methionine; the vitamins B_6, B_{12}, and folic acid; the natural hormone melatonin; and betaine were used, and found to be more effective on GERD and with fewer side effects than the proton pump inhibitor tested (Prilosec).

These supplements were given in the following dosages: 200 milligrams L-tryptophan, 100 milligrams L-methionine, 25 milligrams vitamin B_6, 50 milligrams vitamin B_{12}, 10 milligrams folic acid, 6 milligrams melatonin, and 100 milligrams betaine. According to the study's abstract, "After seven days of supplementation, subjects taking the dietary supplement were found to report relief of symptoms, and after forty days, 100 percent of subjects reported total regression of symptoms."

You can try using these supplements, but may wish to deviate from several of the dosages. The study utilized an unusually high dosage of melatonin, a sleep aid, which probably caused the most common side effect: sleepiness.[32] (It is noteworthy that the subjects also reported better sleep.) The program could be tried with a lower dose of melatonin. (After all, many people get relief from insomnia at just a half milligram of this hormone.) The dosage of folic acid used was more than twelve times what is available in a single pill over the counter in the United States, where the Food and Drug Administration (FDA) limits consumers to 800 micrograms. L-tryptophan is an amino acid and a precursor of the neurotransmitter serotonin, which is used extensively for sleep and mood disorders. Most of the body's serotonin is released in the gut, where it encourages food to move more quickly through the GI system. That would be useful to folks with heartburn, especially if they also experience constipation. Unfortunately, it can be hard to find L-tryptophan supplements in the United States, although it can be found in some health stores. A derivative of L-tryptophan, 5-HTP, is more widely available and should work as well.

The study protocol is safe, does not shut off stomach acid, and appears even more effective than standard drug therapy. Yet I have not been able to find any follow-up studies or news articles. It would be expensive and cumbersome to implement everything exactly as they did in the study, but is possible that lower doses and fewer supplements would achieve the desired the effect (especially in combination with other positive health choices, such as better eating habits).

I would start with a basic supplement program of colostrum, probiotics, and fish oil. I would then add the No Shot B vitamin supplement (listed in the Resource section), which contains vitamin B_{12}, vitamin B_6, and folic acid. If the problem is not solved, try adding the standard label suggestion for 5-HTP. If you are still having heartburn and experience trouble sleeping, add .5 to 1 milligram of melatonin to the regimen.

taking bitters with a meal to see how they affect you because there is the possibility of allergic reaction with virtually any substance. My favorite is Swedish Bitters by NatureWorks.

AbsorbAid

AbsorbAid is a natural product that contains a broad range of enzymes. Unlike most heartburn medications, it brings relief from acid reflux by helping digest the meal rather than blocking acid and stopping digestion. Although the means by which it hurries the meal out of the stomach is perhaps not as efficient as naturally healthy digestion, it is preferred to acid-blocking medications because it at least does not make a low acid situation worse. AbsorbAid is backed by a number of studies that show fringe benefits. These include improved absorption of nutrients such as vitamin B_6, the minerals zinc and selenium, and even omega-3 fatty acids. I prefer the specialized and proven original formula over the newer "Platinum Plus."

Chewable Papaya Tablets

Papaya enzymes help digest proteins. This can often bring relief because undigested protein can delay stomach emptying. American Health makes a product in little rolls you can carry in your pocket. Papaya won't fix a broken digestive system, but it is a safe approach and may cost you less than one dollar to try.

Chamomile Tea

Most of us think of chamomile as relaxing, but it also has an herb lore reputation for soothing the stomach. In Germany, where the government takes herbs very seriously, chamomile has been approved for "gastrointestinal spasms and inflammatory diseases of the gastrointestinal tract." There are no listed side effects or drug interactions. Modern science shows that it helps the stomach by reducing inflammation and improving mucous production. However, don't drink too much chamomile tea because it reduces stomach acid in proportion to the dose.

Prelief

Prelief is a product found in drug stores that works in an interesting way. Rather than reducing the acid in your stomach, Prelief reduces the acid in food and keeps it from burning sensitive tissues. It may be taken internally or added to the food or beverage. This is best used as an occasional and temporary remedy because it does not solve the root cause of your problem. Also, if supplemented continually, this product should be combined with magnesium and other nutrients to assure that the calcium it contains goes into the bones and not elsewhere, causing possible issues, such as kidney stones or bone spurs.

Iberogast

Iberogast, a combination of herbal extracts, is popular in Europe but can be hard to find in the United States. It is, however, available online. Iberogast may protect against ulcers and reduce stomach acidity, without causing rebound acid production.[33] I have no experience with this product, but it might be worth tracking down if you are experiencing acid reflux because you have too much acidity.

Antacids

For very occasional attacks of heartburn for which you need to temporarily neutralize stomach acid, antacids can be helpful in getting the symptoms to subside. I like Milk of Magnesia (MOM), because it does not contain aluminum and is based on the mineral magnesium, for which the body has many uses and of which most Americans have low levels. Therefore, although the product is neutralizing the acid, this fact is somewhat offset by some nutrient value. MOM can have a laxative effect and is not recommended if you have diarrhea. Check with your doctor before using if you are pregnant or on antibiotics, and avoid if you have serious kidney issues.

Slippery Elm

This herb contains mucilage—a substance that can help decrease inflammation—and has a reputation for coating and soothing the digestive tract. If you have excess stomach acid, it can also help by absorbing some of the excess. It is quite safe. Liz Lipski's recipe for Slippery Elm tea instructs to simmer one teaspoon of the bark in two cups of water for twenty minutes, and then strain. Slippery Elm is also available in lozenge form, although this product is usually marketed for scratchy throats.

Marshmallow

Marshmallow is a mucilaginous herb like Slippery Elm. Its mucilage helps with inflammation, soothes mucous membranes, and strengthens digestion. However, it also lowers stomach acid, so marshmallow is not a good choice if you already have low stomach acid.

Homeopathic Remedies

Although quite valued in Europe, India, China, and other parts of the world, homeopathic remedies are not well known in the United States. These are greatly diluted forms of the source material with health properties that are often the exact opposite of what would be experienced if the source material was taken in full strength. At one time, the homeopathic approach was quite popular in the United States. In the early 1900s, however, there was a move to standardize medical practice that caused a squashing of schools of thought such as naturopathy and homeopathy. Yet many of these remedies are consistently being proven effective and safe in modern scientific studies and domestic interest is increasing.

According to expert Dana Ullman, MPH, author of *The Homeopathic Revolution: Why Famous People and Cultural Heroes Choose Homeopathy,* there are several homeopathic remedies that are useful for heartburn. They should be chosen among according to each specific situation. Pulsatilla in homeopathic form may help alleviate indigestion or heartburn after eating fatty food or pork. Ullman says to select this remedy if you are thirsty and don't like stuffy rooms. Nux vomica, on the other hand, is recommended for digestive problems from overeating, stress, or too much alcohol, coffee or medications. That one might be appropriate if you are irritable, impatient, or have a headache that is worse in the morning. Ignatia, an herb that has similar effects to nux vomica, should be considered if the heartburn seems triggered by grief.

Ineffective Products for Heartburn

There are many products that are rumored to be helpful in alleviating the condition of acid reflux. In my experience, however, not all these products are actually useful. I would advise not to use the following products to treat either the cause or symptoms of acid reflux.

Alka-Seltzer: I have not found Alka-Seltzer, the heartburn and indigestion remedy made famous partly due to its catchy "plop, plop, fizz, fizz" slogan and extensive marketing campaigns, to be particularly effective. I would recommend using baking soda instead, as that would provide the same meal-specific acid neutralization without the irritating effects of the aspirin found in Alka-Seltzer.

Mint: Despite its reputation, mint is not recommended for those with acid reflux because it relaxes the LES. However, it is helpful for an upset stomach, diarrhea, and flatulence. The enteric-coated variety supplements are used with success for irritable bowel syndrome. Some after-dinner mint candies may not contain any real mint—but they probably contain plenty of sugar, so you may want to stay away from these, too.

CONCLUSION

As you can see, there are a number of natural remedies worth trying. Yet because these are, for the most part, not patentable substances, there is no economic incentive to do the voluminous studies required for them to be considered "proven" by the standards of the FDA and mainstream medical practice. Even well-studied natural methods and products typically face an uphill approval battle because of medical bias in favor of pharmaceuticals and the drug companies' strong control of communications within the system. Many valid approaches are dismissed as "anecdotal." Personally, I think anecdotes deserve a lot more respect than they receive. They often more accurately reflect the complexities of human variability and real life than studies performed in labs. In many other countries, anecdotes are a driving force behind research.

Whatever methods you try, be consciously observant of any and all effects. You are unique, and will react as such to each product. Fortunately, there is usually a low risk with most natural remedies. They can often be taken right along with conventional approaches, which will allow you to wean off of the medication if your doctor approves. Dosage ranges of natural supplements also tend to be much more forgiving than those of pharmaceuticals, because they don't have the powerful unilateral effects of drugs. Plus, natural remedies, especially the nutritional ones, almost always offer fringe benefits rather than negative side effects. Despite this, you should always check with a knowledgeable health professional or pharmacist before combining medicines and herbs to avoid intensifying or nullifying the desired effects of any component of your program.

CONCLUSION

*"If I'd known I was going to live so long,
I'd have taken better care of myself."*
—LEON ELDRED

Staying up to date on health news can be confusing because there is often so much contradictory information. However, one thing is clear as far as acid reflux is concerned: Taking acid-blocking medications for long periods of time is like playing with a loaded gun. The dire consequences of perpetually low stomach acid, as well as the increased likelihood of side effects the longer these drugs are taken, are reason enough to keep use of acid blockers to a minimum. Further, these medications can allow possibly serious conditions to exist undetected because they cover up the symptoms. Although there *are* rare conditions for which long-term acid blockers may need to be utilized, this small number of patients is not responsible for the tremendous increase in the sale of these medications. Instead, the bulk of patients taking these drugs are first prescribed them and then kept on them indefinitely mainly because the cause of their abdominal pain was never identified and fixed. It is important to remember that we are all different—and therefore need customized solutions.

Stomach acid is *not* evil. However, the condition that is causing the burning symptoms that the acid blockers disguise can be quite serious. It is extremely beneficial to discover why the LES is malfunctioning and/or what is degrading the tissue, as opposed to dealing solely with the pain or evidence of irritation. Ulcers are one condition for which it may be appropriate to temporarily take an acid-blocking medication, because it will give the membranes a break and allow the tissue to heal. Yet, since ulcers can often be healed in a very short time, even these patients should not be on the drugs for long. It is also often possible to heal ulcers without the use of acid-blockers if the situation is not at a critical stage.

There are so many potential causes of heartburn that it is just logical that there is no single "cure" would apply to every case. In fact, the cookie-cutter nature of the conventional approach is one of its greatest drawbacks—and why I emphasize the need to discover which underlying condition you have. Because there may be more than one factor at work, I also recommend starting with the remedies that have the broadest restorative effects.

You may find all the possible root causes daunting if you have yet to discover why you have heartburn, but don't be discouraged. The following step-by-step plan sums up much of the information you have read throughout this book so that you can evaluate and treat your own situation.

1. Get a complete and accurate diagnosis. Regardless of whether your heartburn pain is being addressed by a doctor, chances are you will not achieve long-term healing if you don't know what the underlying problem is. In Chapter 2, we discussed causes of pain including ulcers, *H. pylori*-related gastritis, gallbladder disease, and cancer. These conditions need all be ruled out before a treatment is prescribed. Your physician can check for a hiatus hernia, evaluate the adequacy of your stomach acid to determine whether your levels are low or high, and determine if you have an *H. pylori* infection. Your doctor, chiropractor, or nutritionist can order an ALCAT food sensitivity test to simplify the process of determining which foods may be a source of trouble for you. Your doctor can also tell you if there has been any erosion of your esophagus.

Be alert to other indirect ways your doctor can help. For example, if your physician has prescribed a non-steroidal anti-inflammatory drug (NSAID), you can request a pain reliever that is less harmful to your GI tract. You should also consider finding a natural solution for the cause of the pain for which the NSAID was prescribed.

Do not abruptly stop taking an acid blocker. Sudden changes can confuse the body and cause a rebound reaction. Always tell your doctor that you wish to get off it first. Let him or her know that you wish to attempt to solve the original problem that caused your heartburn rather than using the medication as a crutch. If you have tissue that needs to be healed, you might have to wait a short time to get off the drug. If you are on a proton-pump inhibitor (PPI), you may want to request a short-term change to one of the older H_2 blockers because they are less likely to cause rebound acid production.

2. Change what you eat immediately. Even while waiting for your doctor appointment, you should make the following simple but important changes. Your doctor will not be likely to object to any of them because they all improve general health.

- Eat smaller meals.

- Eat slowly and chew thoroughly, until the food is almost liquid.

- Cut down on unnecessary junk carbohydrates such as sugars and white flour.

- Use herbs and spices in your cooking. They help gut function and overall health in several ways.

- See if eating more raw foods reduces your heartburn.

- Don't mix fruit juices, sweet fruits, and refined starches with meats and heavy food.

- Don't wash your food down with a lot of liquid.

- Avoid trans fats found in partially hydrogenated oils

- Eat more fish and switch to grass fed beef to improve your intake of the anti-inflammatory omega-3 fatty acids.

- Switch your cooking oil to macadamia nut or olive oil to reduce your intake of pro-inflammatory omega-6 fatty acids.

- Watch extremes of salt intake. Too much salty food may lead to heartburn. There is also some concern that an extremely low-salt diet might reduce our capacity to make stomach acid.

- If you are able to do so, select organic meats and produce to avoid the pesticide residues that upset intestinal balance and put your health at risk in many other ways. The following fruits and vegetables are thought to be the most contaminated when from conventional, non-organic sources: apples, bell peppers, celery, cherries, imported grapes, nectarines, peaches, pears, potatoes, red raspberries, spinach, and strawberries.

- Stop eating foods and drinking beverages that burn as they go down. You may be able to add these back when you find out why they were burning and/or you heal the tissue.

3. Change certain habits. This can be extremely beneficial in your quest to reduce acid reflux. Some of these are listed here. For more suggestions, see Chapter 9.

- Stop smoking. There is at least some evidence that it may cause heartburn—and it of course causes lung cancer and heart disease, as well as many other problems.

- Eat dinner in the early evening so that the food is completely digested before you lay down.

- Elevate the head of your bed about 6 inches. This will limit acid from entering your esophagus, although it does not address the root cause of the problem.

- Exercise, because it is associated with lowered risk. However, do not exercise vigorously or lift weights within a couple of hours after meals.

- Drink more water, which will help with detoxification and hunger. Drink it between meals so as not to water down the digestive juices.

4. Take supplements. Start with those listed below because they are fundamental and affect the broadest range of health issues. This list is also helpful for replacing what might have been depleted by either acid blockers or a chronic low acid condition. In fact, all family members—whether or not they have a known digestive issue—can benefit from following this advice.

- Multi-vitamin/mineral. Choose a health food store brand to assure more meaningful doses, more absorbable forms, and to avoid unnecessary manufacturing ingredients.

- Probiotics. For the best effect on all your friendly organisms, choose a product containing live bacteria rather than dried, its own food supply, and natural substances to improve the gut environment.

- Colostrum. For the best potency and value, choose one certified as "First Collection Colostrum."

- Fish oil. Select for freshness and the absence of heavy metal contamination.

5. Carefully consider and research your symptoms using the

methods of analysis listed below. The information you gather will help your doctor support your recovery and narrow down the root cause. These options are free and can save you money on expensive tests because you will have a much better idea of what your doctor should be testing.

- Review the list on page 54 to determine whether you fit the profile for low stomach acid. If you do, you can be tested or do a trial of the habits and supplements that boost acid.

- If you have symptoms of a hiatus hernia (listed on pages 54 to 55), your doctor or body work professional can confirm that diagnosis. A chiropractor or other body work professional can help rectify the situation. I also recommend that you implement the dietary and supplement suggested throughout this book to help heal any damage and strengthen your structure.

- Take the questionnaire on page 218 to see if you may have yeast overgrowth. If you get a high score—which is *not* a good thing in this particular test—follow the diet guidelines in Chapter 8 and the supplement guide in Chapter 11.

- Keep a food/symptom diary for two weeks. It will help you sort out and identify foods, beverages, and situations that cause you pain. It may also reveal foods to which you are sensitive.

- If you think you have problem foods but aren't sure which ones they are, do an elimination diet. Basic instructions were covered in Chapter 9.

- If you don't feel motivated to do the sensitivity research such as a food/symptom diary, go with the odds: Try an enzyme and probiotic supplement, while temporarily eliminating the most common allergens: milk, eggs, peanuts, tree nuts, fish, shellfish, wheat, and soy.

Heartburn Symptom Relief

Although not necessarily a good long-term solution, on-the-spot relief from burning symptoms can be both important and practical. When you first feel the burning sensation, take a few sips of water to flush the digestive juice from the irritated tissue. However, drinking more than a few sips will increase the volume of your stomach contents and dilute the acid, thus slowing its emptying. After drinking this small amount of water, implement one or more of the following suggestions. These suggestions (which were described in more detail in Chapter 11) are natural and cause few side effects. However, don't allow relief from symptoms to lure you into thinking that the bigger problem has been resolved.

- Chew two or three soft probiotic capsules.

- Chew a chewable deglycyrrhizinated licorice (DGL) tablet.

- Take a combination digestive enzyme/HCl capsule. If this helps your situation, check out the supplement recommendations for people with low stomach acid, which is listed on page 213.

- Take a swig of herbal bitters or a spoonful of vinegar in water. If either of these help your situation, check out the supplement recommendations for people with low stomach acid, which is listed on page 213.

- Chew papaya enzymes or swallow a multiple enzyme product.

- Drink 2 ounces of aloe vera.

- For a particularly acute occasional burn or if taking one of the above supplements burns, put a teaspoon of baking soda in water and swallow. This will flush juices off of the tender tissues and neutralize the acid.

6. Once you have determined the root cause of your heartburn, take supplements related to your specific problem.

If you have low stomach acid:

- Make sure you know whether or not *H. pylori* is interfering with your acid production. See the section regarding that bacterium on page 214.

- Lighten the load on stomach acid by eating less heavy protein, chewing more thoroughly, and supplementing with digestive enzymes.

- Stimulate acid production with bitters or vinegar.

- Carefully (and preferably with your doctor's approval and supervision) begin adding betaine HCl supplements.

If your heartburn is related to inflammation (which it is):

- Eat less sugar and trans fats.

- Eat more fruits and vegetables.

- Eliminate foods to which you are sensitive.

- Implement the changes listed in the sections "2. Change what you eat immediately" on page 208, "3. Change certain habits" on page 208, and "4. Take supplements" on page 210.

- Use natural anti-inflammatory substances such as turmeric and ginger (but do so with care).

If you have ulcers or tissue erosion:

- Take Zinc-Carnosine supplements to speed your healing.

- Take deglycyrrhizinated licorice (DGL), which improves and protects the lining of the GI tract.

- Drink aloe vera juice or colostrum, which helps healing.

If your intestinal yeast has become overgrown:

The following bullet points represent the research and advice of visionary Dr. Jeffrey Bland. Although his program, called the "Four Rs," was developed years ago, his advice is still the best regarding yeast overgrowth.

- *Remove* the offending substances (such as allergic foods, NSAIDs, and anything that kills friendly bacteria).

- *Replace* acid, if needed, and enzymes.

- *Reinoculate* supplement probiotics and feed them with pre-biotics.

- *Regenerate* the lining of the intestinal tract with Zinc-Carnosine, DGL, colostrum, the basic nutrients discussed in Chapter 11, and perhaps L-glutamine.

If you have H. pylori:

The only way to confirm the presence of *H. pylori* is with a medical test. However, studying the list of symptoms on page 80 will give you an idea if you should be tested. Key nutritional support for reducing the *H. pylori* bug and healing the damage done includes the following.

- Supplement with DGL, Zinc-Carnosine, Dr. Ohhira's Probiotic 12 Plus probiotics, mastic, turmeric (as a spice and/or supplement), colostrum, and/or berberine.

- You likely have reduced stomach acid; if you do, follow the instructions in the section on page 213 regarding low stomach acid.

- Eat more broccoli, cauliflower, cabbage, and kale. If you are on a medication such as a blood thinner, be sure to notify your doctor of this dietary change.

- Follow the suggestions on page 213 regarding inflammation.

If you must continue taking acid blockers:

If you have to continue taking an acid blocker, there are some actions you can take to offset some of the likely resulting damage.

- Consume easy-to-digest protein sources, such as meal replacement drinks which contain whey protein.
- Take the foundation nutrients listed in "4. Take supplements" on page 210.
- Take enzymes.
- Take a vitamin B_{12}/B_6/folic acid sublingual.
- Take a bone formula with plenty of magnesium.
- Take zinc (if your multi-mineral and bone formula don't contain a combined 15 to 30 milligrams of this nutrient).
- Keep an eye on your iron levels to make sure you do not become anemic.

7. Take other steps to improve your overall health and, likely, your digestion. If you are overweight, you may find that your digestion will improve as you lose weight. At the same time, the yeast-defeating diet described in Chapter 7 is likely to help you lose weight as it eliminates a lot of insulin-raising, craving-producing foods like sugars and starches.

As a country, we need only look at the effect on the economy of soaring sickness care costs and at our plummeting international rank in most health indexes to confirm that we are simply not doing enough to prevent chronic disease. Studies also show that, collectively, Americans could save billions of dollars every year if we incorporated the proper usage of dietary supplements and an integrative approach that included both naturopathic and homeopathic methods. Average citizens can help. We can vote for change by electing legislators who believe that the country should begin studying prevention of disease—rather than just offering a new idea about who should pay for the crisis. We can also vote with our dollars by supporting those professionals and companies that are working for safer, more effective solutions.

However, most of us don't have the time to wait for the whole system to change or for scientific advancements. There are some personal health issues we need to address ourselves. People with chronic heartburn continue to suffer because of the tendency of conventional treatment to concentrate on symptom relief rather than safe and less expensive approaches that deal with the root cause. Rely on your common sense. If you had a thorn in your foot, I hope you would remove the thorn as opposed to taking a painkiller. Similarly, it is always in your best interest to treat the root cause of your heartburn, even if also acting to relieve the symptoms. The lasting solution to your problem is unlikely to come from high-tech drugs and surgery. In fact, there is a very good chance that you already have access to products that can help you.

We can hope that the outlook of our physicians continues to broaden. However, as patients, we will always share the responsibility for our own health. Stay informed of possible causes, be observant of signs, and remain open to new ideas. Most importantly, consistently make healthful choices. After all, we are the sum total of *all* that we do. Every positive and healthy action we take has the potential to help us; every negative and unhealthy action we take adds an insult to the accumulated damage. Of course, it takes determination to implement healthful decisions and nothing is harder than changing our eating habits, but you can at least start slowly with a single step. It will become easier to add additional steps once you begin to see how much better you feel.

The natural approaches offered in this book can help solve your gastrointestinal problem, but they also offer fringe benefits for your whole body and improve your health and vitality for the rest of your life. They are well worth the effort and a little out-of-pocket expense. I wish you the best of luck and good health!

CANDIDA QUESTIONNAIRE

Complete this comprehensive questionnaire to determine if your health problems are likely related to an overgrowth of yeast. The score will give you a general idea as to whether yeast may be your problem. When I suspect a client may have a yeast problem, I use these questions as I make a diagnosis. I adapted and updated them from a questionnaire contained in *The Yeast Connection Handbook* by William G. Crook, MD. Instructions on how to score as well as interpret your responses appear after the questionnaire. Scores for men and women are listed separately because women tend to receive slightly higher scores than men, as seven items in the questionnaire apply exclusively to women, while only two apply exclusively to men.

If you determine that your health issues may be related to yeast, I highly recommend Dr. Crook's book. In addition, read Chapter 8, which describes different remedies for Candida, and the Resource section, which lists more comprehensive sources regarding recommended diet and medications. If symptoms persist after trying these methods, consult your healthcare provider.

CANDIDA QUESTIONNAIRE

HISTORY

The following questions address factors that promote the growth of Candida albicans and are frequently found in people with yeast-related health problems. If you answer "yes" to a question, circle the score that appears next to it.

1. At any time in your life, have you taken tetracyclines or other antibiotics for acne for one month or longer?   35

2. At any time in your life, have you taken broad-spectrum antibiotics or other antibacterial medication for respiratory, urinary, or other infections for two months or longer, or for shorter periods but four or more times in a one-year period?   35

3. At any time in your life, have you taken a broad-spectrum antibiotic drug, even in a single dose?   6

4. At any time in your life, have you been bothered by persistent prostatitis, vaginitis, or other problems affecting your reproductive organs?   25

5. Are you bothered by memory or concentration problems? Do you sometimes feel spacey?   20

6. Do you feel "sick all over" but no cause has been found by your physician?   25

7. Have you been pregnant two or more times?   5

8. Have you been pregnant one time only?   3

9. Have you taken birth control pills for more than two years?   15

10. At any time in your life, have you taken birth control pills for between six months and two years?   8

11. At any time in your life, have you taken steroids—orally, injected, or inhaled—for more than two weeks? 15

12. At any time in your life, have you taken steroids— orally, injected, or inhaled—for two weeks or less? 6

13. Do perfumes, insecticides, fabric shops, and other chemicals provoke moderate to severe symptoms? 20

14. Do perfumes, insecticides, fabric shops, and other chemicals provoke mild symptoms? 5

15. Does tobacco smoke bother you a lot? 10

16. Are your symptoms worse either on damp, muggy days or in moldy places like basements or barns? 20

17. At any time in your life, have you had severe or persistent athlete's foot, ring worm, jock itch, or other chronic fungus infections of the skin or nails? 20

18. At any time in your life, have you had mild to moderate athlete's foot, ring worm, jock itch, or other chronic fungus infections of the skin or nails? 10

19. Do you crave sugar and/or starch? 10

Total of all points circled in Section A _____

MAJOR SYMPTOMS

These symptoms are often present in people with yeast-related health problems. For each of the symptoms in this section, check the appropriate column indicating your experience. If you have not experienced the symptom at all, make no mark. After going through the list, add up the check marks in each column. Then multiply these amounts by the number indicated in the row designated "Points assigned to each column."

Symptoms	Occasional or Mild	Frequent or Moderately Severe	Severe or Disabling
Abdominal pain			
Attacks of anxiety or crying			
Bloating, belching, or intestinal gas			
Constipation and/or diarrhea			
Cramps and/or other menstrual irregularities			
Cystitis (urinary tract infection) or interstitial cystitis			
Depression or manic depression			
Endometriosis or infertility			
Fatigue or lethargy			
Feeling of being "drained"			
Headache			
Heartburn, acid reflux			
Hypothyroidism (symptoms of which include thinning hair, dry skin, fatigue, weight gain, cold hands or feet, and low body temperature)			
Impotence			
Loss of sexual desire or feeling			

Symptoms	Occasional or Mild	Frequent or Moderately Severe	Severe or Disabling
Muscle aches			
Muscle weakness or paralysis			
Numbness, burning, or tingling			
Pain and/or swelling in joints			
Premenstrual tension			
Shaking or irritable when hungry			
Troublesome vaginal burning, itching, or discharge			
Total marks in each column			
Points assigned to each column	x 3	6	9
Product of multiplying above two rows	____ +	____ +	____

Total of all columns in Section B   ____

OTHER SYMPTOMS

These symptoms are sometimes seen in people with yeast-related problems, but can also be caused by other conditions. For each of the symptoms in this section, put a check mark in the appropriate column indicating your experience. If you have not experienced the symptom, make no mark. After going through the list, add up the marks in each column. Then multiply these amounts by the number indicated in the row designated "Points assigned to each column."

Symptoms	Occasional or Mild	Frequent or Moderately Severe	Severe or Disabling
Bad breath			
Burning on urination			
Burning or tearing eyes			
Chronic hives (urticaria)			
Cough or recurrent bronchitis			
Dizziness/loss of balance			
Drowsiness, including inappropriate drowsiness			
Dry mouth or throat			
Ear pain or deafness			
Eczema, itching eyes			
Foot, hair, or body odor that is not relieved by washing			
Frequent mood swings			
Indigestion or heartburn			
Insomnia			
Irritability			
Laryngitis, loss of voice			
Mouth rashes, including "white" tongue			
Mucus in stools			
Nasal congestion or postnasal drip			
Nasal itching			

Symptoms	Occasional or Mild	Frequent or Moderately Severe	Severe or Disabling
Pain or tightness in chest			
Poor coordination			
Pressure above ears/ feeling of head swelling			
Psoriasis			
Rectal itching			
Recurrent ear infections or fluid in ears			
Sensitivity to milk, wheat, corn or other common foods			
Sinus problems/tenderness of cheekbones or forehead			
Sore throat			
Spots in front of eyes or erratic vision			
Tendency to bruise easily			
Urinary frequency or urgency			
Wheezing or shortness of breath			
Total marks in each column			
Points assigned to each column	x 1	2	3
Product of multiplying above two rows	___ +	___ +	___

Total of all columns in Section C ___

In the boxes indicated below, put your scores from Sections A, B, and C. Then add these three numbers together to get your Grand Total.

Total Scores Section A: _____

Section B: _____

Section C: _____

Grand Total: _____

Women

- 180 and up: yeast-related health problems are almost certainly present.

- 120 to 179: yeast-related health problems are probably present.

- 60 to 119: yeast-related health problems are possibly present.

- 59 or lower: yeasts are not likely to be the cause of health problems.

Men

- 140 and up: yeast-related health problems are almost certainly present.

- 90 to 139: yeast-related health problems are probably present.

- 40 to 89: yeast-related health problems are possibly present.

- 39 or lower: yeasts are not likely to be the cause of health problems.

Glossary

Words that appear in *italics* are defined within this glossary.

acid excess. A fairly rare condition in which the stomach contains a high level of hydrochloric acid; usually caused by a tumor in the pancreas or small intestine. See also *heartburn*.

acid indigestion. A digestive disorder caused by excessive stomach acid.

acid reflux. The regurgitation of stomach acid into the esophagus. See also *GER*, *GERD*, *heartburn*, or *NERD*.

acid-blocking drugs. Any medication—including proton pump inhibitors, H_2-receptor antagonists, and antacids—that interferes with the production or process of stomach acid.

acid-suppressing drugs. See *acid-blocking drugs*.

alkaline. Any substance with a *pH* balance higher than 7; the opposite of acid.

amino acids. The building blocks of proteins; commonly known as "aminos." They are components of muscles, neurotransmitters, and hair, as well as most other parts of the body. Despite their name, most of them are neutral rather than acidic.

amylase. A class of enzyme that digests starch.

antacid. An alkaline substance that neutralizes stomach acid. These drugs are typically sold over the counter. They are also shorter acting and safer than the newer classes of acid-blocking drugs. They do not pose much health risk if used occasionally, but the risks increase dramatically when they are used chronically.

antibiotic. A substance that kills bacteria. Although this can include fungus and parasites, the term is typically used to refer to anti-bacterial drugs. They are not effective against viruses. Although a few antibiotics have a narrow range of action, common ones are broad spectrum and kill friendly bacteria along with the pathogenic ones. See also *antibiotic-resistant*.

antibiotic-resistant. Term used to describe an organism that changes so that an antibiotic is no longer effective at killing it. This threat has been growing due to the overuse of antibiotics.

antioxidant. A substance that can protect the body from the harmful effects of *free radicals*. Smoking, radiation, chemicals, and even exercise increase free radicals. Antioxidants—which can be vitamins, minerals, enzymes, or phytonutrients—protect us from them.

Barrett's esophagus. A condition in which the esophagus contains abnormal cells. It is caused by chronic exposure to stomach acid and can lead to cancer.

Candida. A type of yeast that can cause serious symptoms and health problems. There are many aspects of modern life that can allow Candida to become overgrown; the most common is the overuse of antibiotics. These medications damage the colonies of protective bacteria, which otherwise keep yeasts under control. Yeast overgrowth can be difficult to diagnose in the typical medical office, because the symptoms are often subtle and varied, and may be seemingly unrelated to the gut.

celiac disease. An autoimmune digestive disease also known as celiac and sprue. This condition has been underdiagnosed and is associated with bone thinning and many other symptoms.

cellulase. *Enzymes* that digest the cellulose in plant foods. People do not make this type of enzyme; instead, they depend upon *probiotics* to break down plant cells so that we can benefit from its nutrients, including cellulase. The digested fiber feeds the cells lining our intestinal tract.

Complimentary and Alternative Medicine (CAM). Healthcare outside of conventional treatment. According to Harvard Medical School, the most commonly used CAM therapies use herbs, relaxation techniques, and/or chiropractic techniques. See also *integrative medicine*.

conventional medicine. Common medical practice that focuses heavily on the suppression of symptoms rather than determining root causes. This practice often departmentalizes the body, sending each section of a person to a specialist. This is in contrast to *naturopathic medicine* and *homeopathic medicine*.

die-off reaction. Symptoms—including headache, fatigue, or flu—that can occur when bacteria or yeasts are killed off in large numbers and dump their toxic residue into circulation. This can be worsened if the person's detoxification pathways are not clear. Clogged pathways can be indicated by constipation, dehydration, lack of exercise, and having most of the skin covered with creams.

dysbiosis. A condition in which the intestinal bacteria and *yeasts* have become imbalanced in favor of disease-causing organisms. Dysbiosis can result in *leaky gut*.

dyspepsia. An umbrella term that refers to pain or an uncomfortable feeling in the midsection.

elimination diet. A do-it-yourself method of identifying *food sensitivities*. Foods commonly eaten are eliminated for several days, and then added back one at a time while reactions are observed.

enzyme. A catalyst that helps a chemical transaction take place but does not participate in the change. In digestion, enzymes break down foods into smaller units to facilitate absorption.

erosion. Term used to describe tissue that is highly inflamed and irritated. If the erosion causes a hole in the tissue, it is called an *ulcer*.

erosive esophagitis. See *erosive reflux disease*.

erosive reflux disease (ERD). An inflammation of the *esophagus* wherein tissues are seriously damaged. Healing can be quick if you stop doing what caused the problem and use healing supplements. The conventional treatment is to instead stop the production of *stomach acid*.

esophagitis. Any inflammation, swelling, or irritation of the *esophagus*. It commonly occurs with *acid reflux* and often involves pain on swallowing.

esophagus. The muscular tube that connects the throat with the stomach. It is not lined with mucous-secreting cells because it is not supposed to be exposed to acid; therefore, acid backing up into the esophagus can cause pain. See also *lower esophageal sphincter.*

flora. A collection of microorganisms, such as those that line the intestinal tract.

fluoride. A highly toxic industrial waste material added to drinking water because of the unproven justification that it prevents tooth decay. This practice is banned in many countries—although not the United States—because of numerous adverse health effects.

food allergy. A negative reaction by your immune system to a food. Food allergies are typically inherited and the reactions can be quite severe. See also *food sensitivity* and *food intolerance.*

Food and Drug Administration (FDA). US government agency charged with protecting Americans from dangerous and unproven drugs and food contamination.

food intolerance. An inability to digest a particular food or one of its components.

food sensitivity. A negative reaction to food. It is usually acquired as a result of poor maintenance of the intestinal tract membranes, which is typically caused by an overgrowth of yeast.

free radicals. Highly reactive unstable molecules that can start a chain reaction and damage cells; also known as oxidants.

fringe benefits. A positive result of a medication or supplement that is not the reason for which it was taken. Fringe benefits are most often enjoyed with natural approaches, whereas *side effects* are usually experienced with medication.

fungus. Parasitic organisms that are somewhere between plant and animal. Fungus includes those that cause athlete's foot and dandruff as well as intestinal yeast that can overtake the intestinal tract and cause a myriad of symptoms.

gallbladder disease. The gallbladder is a sack that holds and concentrates bile coming from the liver and going into the digestive tract. Gallbladder disease occurs when stones form or infection sets in. Both can cause terrible pain and digestive distress, which is at times confused with *heartburn.*

gastric acid. See *stomach acid.*

gastritis. An inflammation of the stomach membranes. Often caused by *non-steroidal anti-inflammatory drugs (NSAIDs)* or infection by the bacterial strain *H. pylori.*

gastrointestinal reflux (GER). The regurgitation of digestive fluid into the esophagus. GER is quite common. If the condition worsens, it is called *GERD.*

gastroesophageal reflux disease (GERD). Chronic (occurring two to three times a week or for three or more months) regurgitation of digestive fluid into the esophagus. GERD can cause a sore throat or hoarseness.

gastrointestinal (GI). The entire digestive system, from the mouth to the anus.

gluten enteropathy. See *celiac disease.*

gut. Shortterm for gastrointestinal area, usually referring to the intestines.

H. pylori. A strain of bacteria that can cause gastritis and ulcers. It is associated with greatly increased risk of stomach and colon cancer, and is also a suspect in pancreatic cancer and heart disease. It appears along with other conditions such as rosacea, migraine headaches, a type of arthritis, anemia, B$_{12}$ deficiency, glaucoma, bad breath, asthma, and morning sickness.

heartburn. Pain or burning just below the breastbone or in the chest, throat, or jaw caused by the regurgitation of *stomach acid* into the *esophagus*. Symptoms can be confused with asthma. The term is used nearly interchangeably with *GERD*.

histamine receptor antagonists. A class of drugs that stops acid production, although not as effectively or for as long a time as the *PPIs*. Tagamet, Zantac, Mylanta, and Pepcid AC are histamine receptor antagonists. Also known as H$_2$ blockers.

homeopathic medicine. A system of non-toxic but effective medicine used widely in Europe. These substances are regulated by the *Food and Drug Administration* and sold over the counter.

hydrochloric acid (HCl). A major component of *stomach acid*.

immune system. The cells and organs that make up the body's entire defense system.

indigestion. Nearly any kind of unsettled feeling in the stomach after meals; may include some nausea or bloating. Indigestion is the lay equivalent of the term *dyspepsia*.

insurance reimbursement. Payment by insurance company for medical or drug expense. Unfortunately, this often determines what kind of medicine your doctor practices.

integrative medicine. A combination of *conventional medicine* and the "alternative" natural medicine world. This practice is more popular—and successful—in industrialized countries other than the United States.

lower esophageal sphincter (LES). The muscular ring that allows food to proceed to the stomach and keeps stomach juices from backing up into the *esophagus*. Certain conditions cause a weakening of this muscle, allowing it to stay open and *stomach acid* to re-enter the esophagus.

mainstream medicine. See *conventional medicine*.

mucus. A slippery substance made by the mucous membranes in the body. It contains immune factors and enzymes that kill bugs. (It is called phlegm when in the respiratory system.)

mycotoxin. A toxin (poison) produced by a member of the fungus kingdom. Mycotoxins can be found on crops or in the form of an *antibiotic*. They can also be made by *yeasts* inside the *gut*.

Myopractor. A professional who is trained to achieve structural balance by releasing the tension in soft tissue such as muscles, tendons, and fascia. Also known as a body work practitioner. Myopractics is a small but growing field.

naturopathic medicine. A healthcare system that concentrates on keeping a body healthy and how to use natural methods for healing. Nutrition, herbs, homeopathy, midwifery, colon hygiene, and more are utilized. Unfortunately, only a limited number of states have licensed these skilled physicians.

neurotransmitter. A chemical the body makes to send nerve impulses throughout the body.

nonerosive reflux disease (NERD). A form of *GERD* in which the tissue has not yet begun to erode.

non-steroidal anti-inflammatory drugs (NSAIDs). Medications that reduce inflammation but can cause risky side effects, such as ulcers. Examples of common NSAIDs are Aleve, Aspirin, Celebrex, Feldene, ibuprofen, Indocin, Motrin, Naprosyn, and Naproxen.

omega-3 fatty acid. An essential fatty acid that has anti-inflammatory properties and is protective against a number of chronic diseases. The best known source is fish oil.

omega-6 fatty acid. An essential fatty acid that should be consumed in moderation. If eaten in excess, omega-6 fatty acids overpower the *omega-3 fatty acids* and act in a pro-inflammatory way. Omega-6s contain an important metabolite, GLA, that is anti-inflammatory and helpful with problems in many areas such as skin, joints, and PMS. GLA can be taken as a supplement.

osteopenia. Decrease in bone density that can lead to *osteoporosis*.

osteoporosis. Decrease in bone density that can result in weakened and broken bones. Low *stomach acid,* including that caused by *acid-blocking drugs,* interferes with the absorption of calcium and other nutrients needed to build bones.

pancreas. An organ and a gland. It is the source of many digestive substances as well as hormones.

pancreatin. A mixture of enzymes produced by the *pancreas.*

parasite. An organism that lives in the body and feeds off the body's nutrition. They can be single cells or even worms. Parasites can cause diarrhea, nausea, *heartburn,* vomiting, gas and bloating, foul-smelling stools, weight loss, chills, headache, constipation, and fatigue.

pH. A measure of a substance's acidity and alkalinity. The number seven indicates neutrality between the two.

placebo. When the mere perception that an action has been taken causes results. Although often referred to disparagingly, the placebo effect actually shows the power of the mind/body connection. The mind can cause the cells to take an action that can in fact help the situation.

prebiotics. Food for *probiotics.* They are often only fiber, but can also be fruits, vegetables, herbs, and seaweeds.

probiotics. Friendly bacteria (and at least one or two benign yeasts) that live in the intestinal tract and perform a multitude of supportive functions such as protecting the body from harmful bacteria and *yeasts,* making vitamins, digesting foods, nourishing the intestinal membranes, helping to balance hormones, and detoxifying harmful substances. Probiotics are subject to damage from medications, particularly *antibiotics;* poor diet; stress; and the presence of chlorine and fluoride in water.

protease. An enzyme that digests proteins.

proton pump inhibitors (PPIs). Medications that completely halt the production of stomach acid. These include Nexium, Prevacid, Prilosec, Protonix, and AcipHex. Package inserts instruct consumers to use PPIs for no longer than fourteen days but many people unwisely stay on them indefinitely.

rotation diet. A food plan in which a span of four days passes between consumption of the same food product. It minimizes the effects of *food sensitivities* and allows the body to recover from an exposure.

serotonin. A *neurotransmitter* that helps regulate mood, sleep, and appetite. Most of the production of and receptors for serotonin are found in the intestinal tract, not the brain.

side effects. Negative and unintended consequences of a medication or treatment.

statin drugs. A type of medication used to lower cholesterol. *Heartburn* is a potential side effect.

stomach acid. Digestive juice produced by the stomach; also called gastric acid. It protects us from invading organisms, breaks down food, and begins the digestive process.

sub-clinical. A condition that is quietly generating negative health effects without any obvious symptoms, often allowing it to progress undetected.

trans fats. Damaged fats that cause inflammation and gum up our cellular processes, ultimately causing disease. Trans fats are chiefly found in processed foods and often referred to as "partially hydrogenated fats."

ulcers. Holes in the lining of the digestive track; they are usually in the stomach or small intestine. Ulcers occur when inflammation gets out of control and the integrity of the tissue is eroded, and are often caused by *non-steroidal anti-inflammatory drugs (NSAIDs)* and/or an *H. pylori* bacterial infection. They can be fatal if the bleeding is not stopped or the hole becomes deep enough to allow digestive material to leak into the body. The pain is often temporarily relieved by eating.

villi. Very tiny but important fingerlike projections on the surface of the small intestine that greatly increase the surface area for the absorption of nutrients. These can become flat when the intestine is overgrown with *yeast.*

yeast. A member of the fungus kingdom that can cause serious health issues if allowed to grow out of control in the digestive tract or sinuses. See also *Candida.*

RESOURCES

FINDING PRACTITIONERS
OF INTEGRATIVE MEDICINE

Doctors that are up on the latest natural approaches usually belong to organizations that focus their continuing education on those matters. Visit the following websites to find a doctor in your area. You can also go to your neighborhood health food store and talk to the owner or an employee that has been around for a while. Ask them which practitioners in the area get good reviews from customers.

American College for Advancement in Medicine (ACAM)
www.acamnet.org
Association for doctors (MD or DO) that practice complementary, alternative, and integrative medicine.

American Association of Naturopathic Physicians (AANP)
www.naturopathic.org
Association for doctors of naturopathic medicine (ND), who emphasize disease prevention and optimizing wellness.

American Chiropractic Association (ACA)
www.amerchiro.org
Association for chiropractors, who concentrate on the significance of the spinal column and nervous system to general health and well being.

Cancer Treatment Centers of America (CTCA)
www.cancercenter.com
1-800-615-3055
Association that helps and treats cancer patients by gently blending cutting-edge conventional treatments with support from nutritional and natural medicine, as well as mind/body methods.

ALCAT FOOD SENSITIVITY TESTING

www.alcat.com
1-800-872-5228
Possible reactions that can occur as a result of food sensitivities or intolerances run the gamut from quickened breathing to red ears to exhaustion. ALCAT is a blood test that can determine the foods and chemicals to which you are either allergic or sensitive.

FINDING SUPPLEMENTS, FOOD, AND OTHER PRODUCTS

Most of the products I have mentioned are widely available. Some can even be found in drug and grocery stores. When possible, I recommend buying natural products from a natural foods store to assure that you get the best brand. Products in a "professional line" usually come from a chiropractor, nutritionist, or professional's website.

There are some products that are new or not widely available. I chose many of these brands as sponsors for my radio show because I have set a standard of choosing only the best product in each category. To assure that listeners had access to them, I arranged with Real Food Grocery to stock the following items, as well as products I recommend in the future. This store is located in Texas, but can also be found online. In addition, the staff is available by phone, and will gladly tell your health food store or health professional how to stock the items for your convenience.

Real Food Grocery
1-877-673-2536
www.RealFoodGrocery.com

• Café Sonora Organic coffee.

• Dr. Ohhira's Probiotic 12 Plus. These can also be purchased at www.probiotics12.com.

• Enzymes and other Candida-related products.

• Essential Formulas Brazilian Green Propolis.

• Homeopathic remedy for Candida yeast.

• Jarrow Formulas Mastic Gum 500.

• Jarrow Formulas PepZinGI.

• MacNut Oil.

• No Shot B_{12}/B_6/Folic Acid sublingual.

• PerCoBa Colostrum lozenges, powder, capsules, and liquid extract. These can also be purchased at www.PerCoBa.com.

• Water filter that removes flouride.

• Whey protein drink.

BOOKS

Digestion

Digestive Wellness by Elizabeth Lipski, PhD, CCN; Keats. Provides information on and solutions to many digestive problems, including food sensitivities.

Guess What Came to Dinner: Parasites and Your Health by Ann Louise Gittleman, CNS; Avery. Focuses on illness caused by common parasites; newly updated.

Enzymes: Go With Your Gut by Karen DeFelice; ThunderSnow Interactive. Explores the benefits of enzyme therapy, particularly for children with autism or learning and behavior problems.

Enzymes: What the Experts Know by Tom Bohager; One World Press. Discusses pH balance and the therapeutic use of enzymes for purposes other than digestion.

No More Heartburn: Stop the Pain in 30 Days—Naturally! by Sherry Rogers, MD; Kensington Health. Offers advice on dealing with gastrointestinal issues; includes effects of chemicals, MSG, and the sweetener aspartame.

Ulcer Free by Georges M. Halpern, MD, PhD; Square One Publishers. A must-read for anyone with an ulcer.

Why Stomach Acid Is Good for You by Jonathan V. Wright, MD and Lane Lenard, PhD; M Evans and Company, Inc. Includes scholarly information about digestive chemistry as well as patient histories; also covers asthma and depression.

Candida

The Fungus Link: An Introduction to Fungal Disease Including the Initial Phase Diet by Doug Kaufmann; Mediatrition. By the author of *The Germ that Causes Cancer* and *Infectious Diabetes*.

The Yeast Connection Handbook: How Yeasts Can Make You Feel Sick All Over and the Steps You Need to Take to Regain Your Health by William G. Crook, MD; Square One Publishers. Comprehensive resource on this often-misunderstood health problem.

Other Important Topics

The Hampton's Diet by Fred Pescatore, MD; Wiley. Explains the benefits of and how to eat an Americanized version of the Mediterranean diet.

Lick the Sugar Habit by Nancy Appleton, PhD; Avery Publishing Group Inc. Explains the sources and effects of sugar, and the means to overcome the addiction.

Natural Alternatives to Vioxx, Celebrex, and Other Anti-Inflammatory Prescription Drugs by Carol Simontacchi, MS, CCN; Square One Publishers. A quick and easy read for alternatives to medications that relieve pain and inflammation.

Pain Free in 6 Weeks by Sherry Rogers, MD; Prestige Publishing. A thorough guide to detoxifying, getting to the source of various types of chronic pain, and staying off of NSAIDs.

The Slow Down Diet by Marc David; Health Arts Press. Describes how to reduce your stress, improve your health, and enjoy your life.

General Reference

Consumer Drug Reference by American Society of Health-System Pharmacists; Consumer Reports. Includes everything you need to know about nearly any drug.

Dr. Atkins' Vita-Nutrient Solution: Nature's Answer to Drugs by Robert Atkins, MD; Fireside. Discusses the role and importance of nutritional supplements; with substantial assistance from brilliant nutritionist Robert Crayon.

Encyclopedia of Natural Medicine by Michael T. Murray, ND and Joseph Pizzorno, ND; Prima Health. A wonderfully responsible and comprehensive reference.

Encyclopedia of Nutritional Supplements by Michael T. Murray, ND; Prima. An exhaustive reference on all types of dietary supplements.

Herb Contraindications and Drug Interactions by Francis Brinker, ND; Eclectic Medical Publications. Authoritative manual on combining herbs with medication.

The Homeopathic Revolution: Why Famous People and Cultural Heroes Choose Homeopathy by Dana Ullman, MPH; North Atlantic Books. An entertaining way to learn about and gain confidence in homeopathy.

Supplement Your Prescriptions by Hyla Cass, MD; Basic Health. A guide to utilizing nutrition to avoid drug side effects.

WEBSITES OF INTEREST

Martie Whittekin, CCN website
www.HBNShow.com
Subscribe to Martie's free weekly email newsletter. Site has many free articles, useful links and archives of past programs.

Foundation for Integrative Medicine

http://mdheal.org/leakygut.htm

Information on leaky gut syndrome from Dr. Leo Galland.

The Helicobacter Foundation

www.helico.com

Official H. pylori website that includes information on current treat-ment protocols.

The Price-Pottenger Nutrition Foundation

www.ppnf.org

Offers educational information about food, particularly whole food and preparation, and health.

Total Wellness Newsletter

www.prestigepublishing.com

1-800-846-6687

Monthly newsletter by Sherry Rogers, MD, that includes up-to-date health information.

The Weston A. Price Foundation

www.westonaprice.org

Provides information about food and health; explores these features from a scientific and historical angle.

Fluoride Action Network

www.fluoridealert.org/health

Database of concerns regarding the presence of fluoride in drinking water.

TELEVISION

Know the Cause

Daily health television program hosted by Doug Kaufmann. Visit www.know-the-cause.com to find the show in your area.

References

Chapter 1

1. *J Natl Cancer Inst.* 2005 Jan 19;97(2):142–6. The role of overdiagnosis and reclassification in the marked increase of esophageal adenocarcinoma incidence. Pohl H, Welch HG.

2. *JAMA.* 1998 Apr 15;279(15):1200–5. Incidence of adverse drug reactions in hospitalized patients: a meta-analysis of prospective studies. Lazarou J, et al.

Chapter 2

1. *Aliment Pharmacol Ther.* 2007 Dec 6. Mortality rates in patients with Barrett's oesophagus. Moayyedi P, et al.

2. *Am J Gastroenterol.* 2008 May 20. Dietary antioxidants, fruits, and vegetables and the risk of Barrett's Esophagus. Kubo A, et al.

3. *Nutr Cancer.* 2008 Jan-Feb;60(1):39–48. Dietary supplement use and risk of neoplastic progression in esophageal adenocarcinoma: a prospective study. Dong LM, et al.

4. *Aliment Pharmacol Ther.* 2007 Oct 26. The prevalence and risk factors of erosive oesophagitis and non-erosive reflux disease: a nationwide multi-centre prospective study in Korea. Kim N, et al.

5. *Med Mycol.* 2007 Aug 28;1–7. Chronic mucocutaneous candidiasis and oesophageal cancer. Rosa DD, et al.

6. *Drugs.* 2006;66 Suppl 1:1–5; discussion 29–33. Current understanding of the mechanisms of gastro-oesophageal reflux disease. Orlando RC.

7. *Ann Allergy Asthma Immunol.* 1997 Oct;79(4):333–8. Esophageal candidiasis as a complication of inhaled corticosteroids. Simon MR, et al.

8. *Drugs*. 2006;66 Suppl 1:1–5; discussion 29–33. Current understanding of the mechanisms of gastro-oesophageal reflux disease. Orlando RC.

9. *Aten Primaria*. 2002 Dec;30(10):663–4. Ongoing treatment with omeprazole and appearance of oropharyngeal candidiasis. Pérez Prim FJ, Vila I. [Article in Spanish.]

10. *Am J Gastroenterol*. 1983 May;78(5):261–4. Ketoconazole treatment of Candida esophagitis: a prospective study of 12 cases. Fazio RA, et al.

11. *Aliment Pharmacol Ther*. 2007 Oct 26. The prevalence and risk factors of erosive oesophagitis and non-erosive reflux disease: a nationwide multi-centre prospective study in Korea. Kim N, et al.

12. *Clin Gastroenterol Hepatol*. 2007 Jun;5(6):690–5. Distinct clinical characteristics between patients with nonerosive reflux disease and those with reflux esophagitis. Wu JC, et al.

13. *Fam Med*. 2001 Jul–Aug;33(7):528–32. Speaking and interruptions during primary care office visits. Rhoades DR, McFarland KF, Finch WH, Johnson AO.

14. *Klin Med (Mosk)*. 2006;84(2):71–4. [Hiatus hernia and gastroesophageal reflux disease as a manifestation of a newly revealed hypothyroidism] Savina LV, et al. [Article in Russian.]

Chapter 3

1. *JAMA*. 2006 Dec 27;296(24):2947–53. Long-term proton pump inhibitor therapy and risk of hip fracture. Yang YX, et al.

2. *Clin Nephrol*. 2007 Aug;68(2):65–72. Pump inhibitors and the kidney: critical review. Brewster UC, et al. PMID: 17722704.

3. *Aliment Pharmacol Ther*. 2005 Jul 1;22(1):59–65. Omeprazole delays gastric emptying in healthy volunteers: an effect prevented by tegaserod. Tougas G, et al.

4. *Dig Liver Dis*. 2001 Nov;33(8):707–19. Changes in gastric mucosa and luminal environment during acid-suppressive therapy: a review in depth. Sanduleanu S, et all.

5. *Korean J Gastroenterol*. 2007 Dec;50(6):363–9. The role of gastric

acid in the H. Pylori-induced gastritis in mouse. Kim SS, et al. [Article in Korean.]

6. *J Am Geriatr Soc.* 2007 Aug;55(8):1248–53. The association between cognition and histamine-2 receptor antagonists in African Americans. Boustani M, et al.

7. *N Engl J Med.* 2007 Dec 20; 357(25):2636–2637. Gynecomastia. Romao I.

8. *N Engl J Med.* 1989 Aug 3;321(5):269–74. The effects of cimetidine on the oxidative metabolism of estradiol. Galbraith RA, Michnovicz JJ.

9. *Cancer Epidemiol Biomarkers Prev.* 2007 Dec;16(12):2623–30. Dairy products, calcium intake, and risk of prostate cancer in the prostate, lung, colorectal, and ovarian cancer screening trial. Ahn J, et al. for the Prostate, Lung, Colorectal, and Ovarian Trial Project Team.

10. *Clin Pharmacol Ther* 1998; 63: 397–402. Grapefruit juice greatly increases serum concentrations of lovastatin and lovastatin acid. Kantola T, et al.

Chapter 4

1. *Am J Clin Nutr.* 2007 Aug;86(2):434–43. High folate intake is associated with lower breast cancer incidence in postmenopausal women in the Malmö Diet and Cancer cohort. Ericson U, et al.

2. *J Natl Cancer Inst.* 2004 Mar 3;96(5):396–402. Dietary folate intake and incidence of ovarian cancer: the Swedish Mammography Cohort. Larsson SC, et al.

3. American Heart Association, "What is Homocysteine?," 2008, www.americanheart.org/presenter.jhtml?identifier=535.

4. *Biochim Biophys Acta.* 2004 May 24;1689(1):13–21. Low magnesium promotes endothelial cell dysfunction: implications for atherosclerosis, inflammation and thrombosis. Maier JA, et al.

5. *Obesity (Silver Spring).* 2007 May;15(5):1139–46. Intake of dietary magnesium and the prevalence of the metabolic syndrome among US adults. Ford ES, et al.

6. *Mol Aspects Med*. 2003 Feb-Jun;24(1-3):39-52. Role of magnesium in insulin action, diabetes and cardio-metabolic syndrome X. Barbagallo M, et al.

7. *Przegl Lek*. 2002;59(4-5):267-8. The importance of determination of magnesium concentration in the serum of patients with cancer metastases to the liver. Kopa_ski Z, et al.

8. *J Nutr*. 2003 Sep;133(9):2879-82. Dietary magnesium intake in a national sample of US adults. Ford ES, Mokdad AH.

9. *Indian J Gastroenterol*. 2002 Nov-Dec;21(6):216-8. Effect of omeprazole on plasma zinc levels after oral zinc administration. Ozutemiz AO, et al.

10. *J Am Col Nutr*. 1991 Aug;10(4):372-5. Inhibition of gastric acid secretion reduces zinc absorption in man. Sturniolo GC, et al.

11. *Ophthalmology*. 2007 Jul 28; [Epub ahead of print] Dietary antioxidants and the long-term incidence of age-related macular degeneration: The Blue Mountains Eye Study. Tan JS, et al.

12. *J Natl Cancer Inst*. 2005 Feb 16;97(4):301-6. Zinc concentration in esophageal biopsy specimens measured by x-ray fluorescence and esophageal cancer risk. Abnet CC, et al.

13. *J Int Med Res*. 2007 Sep-Oct;35(5):692-5. Magnesium, zinc and copper status in osteoporotic, osteopenic and normal post-menopausal women. Mutlu M, et al.

14. *J Am Col Nutr*. 1995 Aug;14(4):364-8. Hypochlorhydria from short-term omeprazole treatment does not inhibit intestinal absorption of calcium, phosphorus, magnesium or zinc from food in humans. Serfaty-Lacrosniere C, et al.

15. *Dig Dis Sci*. 2006 Jan;51(1):84-8. Validation of the blood quininium resin test for assessing gastric hypochlorhydria. De Martel C, et al.

Chapter 6

1. *Lancet*. 2006 Jun 24;367(9528):2086-100. Lancet. 2006 Sep 16;368(9540):986; author reply 986-7. Gastro-oesophageal reflux disease. Moayyedi P, Talley NJ.

2. *J Dig Dis.* 2007 Nov;8(4):203–6. Increased prevalence of Helicobacter pylori infection in gastric cardia of patients with reflux esophagitis: a study from Jordan. Abdul-Razzak KK, Bani-Hani KE.

3. The Helicobacter Foundation, "Epidemiology," 2006, www.helico.com/h_epidemiology.html.

4. *Cell Host Microbe.* 2007 Oct 11;2(4):250–63. Helicobacter pylori dampens gut epithelial self-renewal by inhibiting apoptosis, a bacterial strategy to enhance colonization of the stomach. Mimuro H, et al.

5. *World J Surg Oncol.* 2007 May 12;5:51. Helicobacter pylori in colorectal neoplasms: is there an aetiological relationship? Jones M, et al.

6. *Clin Gastroenterol Hepatol.* 2007 Nov 6; Relationship between helicobacter pylori infection and esophageal neoplasia: a meta-analysis. Rokkas T, et al.

7. *Altern Ther Health Med.* 2005 Sep–Oct;11(5):26–9. Management of dyspepsia and peptic ulcer disease. Ryan SW.

8. *Zh Mikrobiol Epidemiol Immunobiol.* 2007 Mar–Apr;(2):71–5. Microbiocenosis of stomach in children with chronic gastritis. [Article in Russian.]

9. *Ann Intern Med.* 2001 Mar 6;134(5):361–9. Therapy for Helicobacter pylori in patients with nonulcer dyspepsia. A meta-analysis of randomized, controlled trials. Laine L, et al.

10. *Med Decis Making.* 2007 Dec 5 [Epub ahead of print]. A second-order simulation model of the cost-effectiveness of managing dyspepsia in the United States. Barton PM, et al.

11. *Helicobacter.* 2007 Nov;12 Suppl 2:59–63. Role of Probiotics in Patients with Helicobacter Pylori Infection. Franceschi F, et al.

12. *J Appl Bacteriol.* 1995 Oct;79(4):475–9. In vitro inhibition of Helicobacter pylori NCTC 11637 by organic acids and lactic acid bacteria. Midolo PD, et al.

13. *Proc Natl Acad Sci USA.* 2002 May 28;99(11):7610–5. Sulforaphane inhibits extracellular, intracellular, and antibiotic-resistant

strains of Helicobacter pylori and prevents benzo[a]pyrene-induced stomach tumors. Fahey JW, et al.

14. *Antimicrob Agents Chemother.* 2003 Dec;47(12):3982–4. Efficacy of sulforaphane in eradicating Helicobacter pylori in human gastric xenografts implanted in nude mice. Haristoy X, et al.

15. *Dig Dis Sci.* 2005 Nov;50(11):2191–3. Curcumin therapy in inflammatory bowel disease: a pilot study. Holt PR.

16. *World J Gastroenterol.* 2005 Dec 21;11(47):7499–507. Bactericidal and anti-adhesive properties of culinary and medicinal plants against Helicobacter pylori. O'Mahony R, et al.

17. *Helicobacter.* 2007 Jun;12(3):238–43. A curcumin-based 1-week triple therapy for eradication of Helicobacter pylori infection: something to learn from failure? Di Mario F, et al.

18. *Korean J Gastroenterol.* 2007 Dec;50(6):363–9. The Role of Gastric Acid in the H. Pylori-Induced Gastritis in Mouse. Kim SS, et al. [Article in Korean.]

19. *Bottom Line Personal,* 2007 June 21. Soothe Your Stomach Naturally, Without Drugs. Galland L.

20. *N Engl J Med.* 1998 Dec 24;339(26):1946. Mastic gum kills Helicobacter pylori. Huwez FU, et al.

21. *J Appl Microbiol.* 2007 Nov 20. The effect of simulated gastric environments on the anti-Helicobacter activity of garlic oil. O'Gara EA, et al.

22. *Zhonghua Yu Fang Yi Xue Za Zhi.* 2007 Jun;41 Suppl:104–7. Effect of selenium-enriched garlic on chronic gastritis of the glandular stomach of Mongolian gerbils induced by H. pylori. Gu LK, et al.

23. *Hepatogastroenterology.* 2007 Jan-Feb;54(73):320–4. Adjuvant effect of vitamin C on omeprazole-amoxicillin-clarithromycin triple therapy for Helicobacter pylori eradication. Chuang CH, et al.

24. *J Physiol Pharmacol.* 2006 Nov;57 Suppl 5:125–36. Ascorbic acid attenuates aspirin-induced gastric damage: role of inducible nitric oxide synthase. Konturek PC, et al.

25. *Eur J Epidemiol.* 2005;20(1):67–71. Effect modification by vitamin

C on the relation between gastric cancer and Helicobacter pylori. Kim DS, et al.

26. *J Agric Food Chem*. 2007 Sep 5;55(18):7377–86. Inhibition of gastric H(+),K(+)-ATPase and Helicobacter pylori growth by phenolic antioxidants of Curcuma amada. Siddaraju MN, Dharmesh SM.

27. *Epidemiology*. 2001 Mar;12(2):209–14. Alcohol as a gastric disinfectant? The complex relationship between alcohol consumption and current Helicobacter pylori infection. Brenner H, et al.

28. *Helicobacter*. 2007 Nov;12 Suppl 2:50–8. Evolution of Helicobacter pylori Therapy from a Meta-analytical Perspective. Gisbert JP, et al.

29. *Helicobacter*. 2007 Dec;12(6):638–42. Double-Dose, New-Generation Proton Pump Inhibitors Do Not Improve Helicobacter pylori Eradication Rate. Choi HS, et al.

Chapter 7

1. *Aten Primaria*. 2002 Dec;30(10):663–4. Ongoing treatment with omeprazole and appearance of oropharyngeal candidiasis. Pérez Prim FJ, Vila I.

2. *Wiad Lek*. 2002;55(1–2):19–28. Microflora of gastric juice in patients after eradication of Helicobacter pylori and treatment with a proton pump inhibitor. Go_cimski A, et al. [Article in Polish.]

3. *Ann Allergy Asthma Immunol*. 1997 Oct;79(4):333–8. Esophageal candidiasis as a complication of inhaled corticosteroids. Simon MR, et al.

4. *Fortschr Med*. 1981 Feb 5;99(5):123–7. Spectrum of esophagitis: etiology, diagnosis, therapy. Rösch W. [Article in German.]

5. *Dis Esophagus*. 2006;19(3):189–92. A study of candida esophagitis in elderly patients attending a district general hospital in the UK. Weerasuriya N, Snape J.

6. *Med Mycol*. 2007 Aug 28;1–7 Chronic mucocutaneous candidiasis and oesophageal cancer. Rosa DD, et al.

7. *Pathol Res Pract*. 2007;203(10):705–15. Fungal infections of the heart: a clinicopathologic study of 50 autopsy cases. Chinen K, et al.

8. *Pediatrics*. 1999 Dec;104(6):1251–7. Antimicrobial use for pediatric upper respiratory infections: reported practice, actual practice, and parent beliefs. Watson RL, et al.

9. *Nippon Ika Daigaku Zasshi*. 1994 Nov;61(6):563–71. Studies on the relationship between gastric acidity and the development of MRSA. Especially for the prevention of MRSA enterocolitis. Suzuki S. [Article in Japanese.]

10. *J Physiol Pharmacol*. 2006 Nov;57 Suppl 9:35–49. Are probiotics effective in the treatment of fungal colonization of the gastrointestinal tract? Experimental and clinical studies. Zwoli_ska-Wcis_o M, et al.

11. *Pathol Res Pract*. 2007;203(10):705–15. Fungal infections of the heart: a clinicopathologic study of 50 autopsy cases. Chinen K, et al.

12. *Med Hypotheses*. 2001 Nov;57(5):570–2. Does gastrointestinal Candida albicans prevent ubiquinone absorption? Krone CA, et al.

13. *J Microbiol Biotechnol*. 2007 Nov;17(11):1797–804. Damage to the cytoplasmic membrane and cell death caused by lycopene in Candida albicans. Sung WS, et al.

14. *Ceska Gynekol*. 2005 Sep;70(5):395–9. Antifungal effect in selected natural compounds and probiotics and their possible use in prophylaxis of vulvovaginitis. Hronek M. [Article in Czech.]

15. *Yeast*. 2007 Aug;24(8):695–706. Diallyl disulphide depletes glutathione in Candida albicans: oxidative stress-mediated cell death studied by two-photon microscopy. Lemar KM.

16. *Bioorg Med Chem Lett*. 2007 Dec 1;17(23):6417–20. Stereoselective synthesis and cytotoxicity of a cancer chemopreventive naphthoquinone from Tabebuia avellanedae. Yamashita M, et al.

17. *Sidahora*. 1995 Winter;40–1. Natural remedies for vaginal infections. Genet J. [Article in Spanish.]

18. *Microbios*. 1991;67(271):95–105. Protection against Candida albicans gastrointestinal colonization and dissemination by saccharides in experimental animals. Ghannoum MA.

19. *J. Essent. Oil Res*. 1998 Nov-Dec;10 (6); 618–627. Chemical com-

position, antimicrobial and antioxidative activity of laurel, sage, rosemary, oregano and coriander essential oils. Baratta, MT, et al.

20. *J Applied Nutr.* 1995;47:96–102. The inhibition of Candida albicans by oregano. Stiles JC, et al.

21. *Phytother Res.* 2000 May;14(3):213–4. Inhibition of enteric parasites by emulsified oil of oregano in vivo. Force M, et al.

22. Grapefruit Seed Extract: Research Update, Supply Side West Conference 2007, Rob McCaleb, President of Herb Research Foundation.

23. *Am J Gastroenterol.* 1983 May;78(5):261–4. Ketoconazole treatment of Candida esophagitis—a prospective study of 12 cases. Fazio RA, et al.

Chapter 8

1. *Dig Dis Sci.* 2006 Aug;51(8):1307–12. Epub 2006 Jul 27. A very low-carbohydrate diet improves gastroesophageal reflux and its symptoms. Austin GL, et al.

2. US Food and Drug Administration, "Approximate pH of Foods and Food Products," 2008 Feb 20, www.cfsan.fda.gov/~comm/lacf-phs.html.

3. Miami Museum of Science, "The pH Factor," 2001, www.miamisci.org/ph/hhoh.html.

4. Stein Carter, J, "pH Testing Results," 2000 Sept 2, http://biology.clc.uc.edu/scripts/pHResl.pl.

5. *Arch Intern Med.* 2006 May 8;166(9):965–71. Are lifestyle measures effective in patients with gastroesophageal reflux disease? An evidence-based approach. Kaltenbach T, et al.

6. *Clin Gastroenterol Hepatol.* 2007 Apr;5(4):439–44. Epub 2007 Mar 23. The effects of dietary fat and calorie density on esophageal acid exposure and reflux symptoms. Fox M, et al.

7. *Epidemiology.* 2001 Mar;12(2):209–14. Alcohol as a gastric disinfectant? the complex relationship between alcohol consumption and current Helicobacter pylori infection. Brenner H, et al.

8. *Nat Clin Pract Neurol.* 2007 Oct;3(10):581–4. A case of celiac disease mimicking amyotrophic lateral sclerosis. Turner MR, et al.

Chapter 9

1. *Am J Physiol Gastrointest Liver Physiol.* 289: G197–G201, 2005. Inhibition of transient lower esophageal sphincter relaxations by electrical acupoint stimulation. Duowu Zou,et al.

2. *Med Clin North Am.* 1991 Jul;75(4):967–79. Diet and nutrition in ulcer disease. Marotta RB, et al.

3. *Aliment Pharmacol Ther.* 2005 Jul 1;22(1):59–65. Omeprazole delays gastric emptying in healthy volunteers: an effect prevented by tegaserod. Tougas G, et al.

4. *Gut.* 2007 Sep;56(9):1177–80. Stress-related changes in oesophageal permeability: filling the gaps of GORD? Söderholm JD.

5. *Arch Intern Med.* 2006 May 8;166(9):965–71. Are lifestyle measures effective in patients with gastroesophageal reflux disease? an evidence-based approach. Kaltenbach T, et al.

6. *J Prev Med Pub Health.* 2007 Nov;40(6):467–74. Cigarette smoking and gastric cancer risk in a community-based cohort study in Korea. Kim Y, et al.

Chapter 10

1. *J Physiol Pharmacol.* 2006 Nov;57 Suppl 9:35–49. Are probiotics effective in the treatment of fungal colonization of the gastrointestinal tract? Experimental and clinical studies. Zwoli_ska-Wcis_o M, et al.

2. *Curr Pharm Des.* 2005;11(1):75–90. Modulation of the human gut microflora towards improved health using prebiotics—assessment of efficacy. Tuohy KM, et al.

Chapter 11

1. *Nat Med.* 1999 Dec;5(12):1418–23. Inhibition of angiogenesis by nonsteroidal anti-inflammatory drugs: insight into mechanisms and implications for cancer growth and ulcer healing. Jones MK, et al.

2 *Dig Dis Sci.* 2001 Apr;46(4):845–51. Effects of polaprezinc on lipid

peroxidation, neutrophil accumulation, and TNF-alpha expression in rats with aspirin-induced gastric mucosal injury. Naito Y, et al.

3. *Phytother Res.* 2000 Dec;14(8):581–91. The plant kingdom as a source of anti-ulcer remedies. Borrelli F, Izzo AA.

4. *J Pharm Pharmacol.* 1980 Feb;32(2):151. Aspirin-induced gastric mucosal damage in rats: cimetidine and deglycyrrhizinated liquorice together give greater protection than low doses of either drug alone. Bennett A, et al.

5. *Practitioner.* 1973 Jun;210(260):820–3. Deglycyrrhizinated liquorice in duodenal ulcer. Tewari SN, Wilson AK.

6. *Digestion.* Effect of deglycrrhised liquorice compound on the gastric mucosal barrier of the dog. 1974;11:355–363. Morris TJ, et al.

7. *Lancet.* 1982 Oct 9;2(8302):817. Deglycyrrhizinated liquorice for peptic ulcer. Glick L.

8. *Nippon Yakurigaku Zasshi.* 1992 Apr;99(4):255–63.The gastric mucosal adhesiveness of Z-103 in rats with chronic ulcer. Seiki M, et al.

9. *Jpn J Pharmacol.* 1995 Apr;67(4):271–8. Residence time of pola - prezinc (zinc L-carnosine complex) in the rat stomach and adhesiveness to ulcerous sites. Furuta S, et al.

10. *Can J Gastroenterol.* 2002 Nov;16(11):785–9. Inhibitory effect of polaprezinc on the inflammatory response to Helicobacter pylori. Handa O, et al.

11. *Helicobacter.* 2007 Feb;12(1):43–8. Low concentrations of zinc in gastric mucosa are associated with increased severity of Helicobacter pylori-induced inflammation. Sempértegui F, et al.

12. *FEMS Immunol Med Microbiol.* 2006 Dec;48(3):347–54. Epub 2006 Sep 21. Potential prophylactic value of bovine colostrum in necrotiz - ing enterocolitis in neonates: an in vitro study on bacterial attachment, antibody levels and cytokine production. Brooks HJ, et al.

13. *Br J Nutr.* 2000 Nov;84 Suppl 1:S127–34. In vivo antimicrobial and antiviral activity of components in bovine milk and colostrum involved in non-specific defence. Van Hooijdonk AC, et al.

14. *Appl Microbiol Biotechnol.* 2007 Jun;75(3):711. Synergistic antidi-

gestion effect of Lactobacillus rhamnosus and bovine colostrums in simulated gastrointestinal tract (in vitro). Wei H, et al.

15. *Am J Clin Nutr.* 2008 Apr;87(4):949–56. Effect of n-3 polyunsaturated fatty acids on Barrett's epithelium in the human lower esophagus. Mehta SP, et al.

16. *Am J Clin Nutr.* 2004 Sep;80(3):752–8. Higher 25-hydroxyvitamin D concentrations are associated with better lower-extremity function in both active and inactive persons aged > or =60 y. Bischoff-Ferrari HA, et al.

17. *Eur J Epidemiol.* 2005;20(1):67–71. Effect modification by vitamin C on the relation between gastric cancer and Helicobacter pylori. Kim DS, et al.

18. *J Physiol Pharmacol.* 2006 Nov;57 Suppl 5:125–36. Ascorbic acid attenuates aspirin-induced gastric damage: role of inducible nitric oxide synthase. Konturek PC, et al.

19. *Proc Nutri Soc.* Vitamin E and its effect on aspirin induce gastric lesion in rats. Aust 2004, Vol. 28. Jaarin K, et al.

20. *Lancet.* 2000 Nov 4;356(9241):1573–4. Dietary vitamin E, IgE concentrations, and atopy. Fogarty A, et al.

21. *Int J Tissue React.* 1983;5(3):301–7. Cytoprotective effect of vitamin A and its clinical importance in the treatment of patients with chronic gastric ulcer. Patty I, et al.

22. *J Bacteriol.* 2005 Sep;187(17):6128–36. Biodiversity-based identification and functional characterization of the mannose-specific adhesin of Lactobacillus plantarum. Pretzer G, et al.

23. *Microbios.* 1991;67(271):95–105. Protection against Candida albicans gastrointestinal colonization and dissemination by saccharides in experimental animals. Ghannoum MA, et al.

24. *Cal Med.* 70:10–14, 1949. Rapid healing of peptic ulcers in patients receiving fresh cabbage juice. Cheney G.

25. *Tex J Med.* 53; 840–3, 1957. Glutamine in treatment of peptic ulcer. Shive W, et al.

26. *Arch Surg.* 1990 Aug;125(8):1040–5. Oral glutamine accelerates

healing of the small intestine and improves outcome after whole abdominal radiation. Klimberg VS, et al.

27. *J Parenter Enteral Nutr.* 1998 Jul–Aug;22(4):224–7. Glutamine enhances gut glutathione production. Cao Y, et al.

28. *Scand J Gastroenterol.* 1993 Jan;28(1):89–94. Gastroprotective capability of exogenous phosphatidylcholine in experimentally induced chronic gastric ulcers in rats. Dunjic BS, et al.

29. *Gastroenterology.* 1994 Aug;107(2):362–8. Lipids of human gastric mucosa: effect of Helicobacter pylori infection and nonalcoholic cirrhosis. Nardone G, et al.

30. *J Ethnopharmacol.* 2007 Apr 4;110(3):567–71. Effect of Brazilian green propolis on experimental gastric ulcers in rats. De Barros MP, et al.

31. *Asian Pac J Cancer Prev.* 2006 Jan-Mar;7(1):22–31. Biological activity of bee propolis in health and disease. Khalil ML.

32. *Acta Pharm.* 2005 Dec;55(4):423–30. Flavonoid analysis and antimicrobial activity of commercially available propolis products. Kosalec I, et al.

33. *J Pineal Res.* 2006 Oct;41(3):195–200. Regression of gastroesophageal reflux disease symptoms using dietary supplementation with melatonin, vitamins and aminoacids: comparison with omeprazole. Pereira Rde S.

34. *Phytomedicine.* 2006;13 Suppl 5:56–66. Epub 2006 Sep 11. Mechanisms involved in the gastro-protective effect of STW 5 (Iberogast) and its components against ulcers and rebound acidity. Khayyal MT, et al.

ABOUT THE AUTHOR

Martie Whittekin is a Certified Clinical Nutritionist with twenty-five years of experience in the trenches. Today, she is fully devoted to health education. Martie hosts *The Martie Whittekin Show: Healthy by Nature*, a nationally syndicated weekly radio talk show in Dallas, TX, that is now in its eleventh year. She interviews authors, doctors, scientists, and other experts on health, and accepts questions and comments from callers. An eager researcher, Martie is always on the alert for superior health products and uses her radio show as an avenue to share her findings with listeners.

Martie spent six years at Ohio State University, and has since been fortunate enough to study with some of the brightest minds in the natural health field. She served on the Board of Trustees for Bastyr University (a fully accredited school of natural medicine) in Seattle. Martie was honored in 1993 as the Association of Women in Nutrition's (AWIN's) "Woman of the Year." Long a champion of preserving freedom of choice in health, she also served as President of the National Nutritional Foods Association (NNFA) during crucial phases of its effort to pass the Dietary Supplement Health and Education Act. In addition, Martie was a founder and president of Texans for Health Freedom, a group formed to protect a citizen's right to choose alternative medical treatments.

To learn more about Martie Whittekin, visit her website at www.HBNShow.com, like her on Facebook, or follow her on Twitter.

INDEX

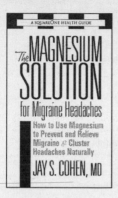
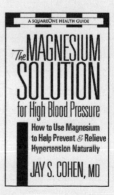

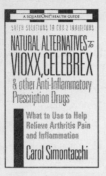
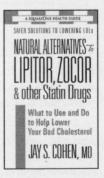